S0-BAU-351

Acclaim for

THE WISDOM TO CHOOSE

"[*The Wisdom To Choose*] counsels that you should prepare a concise summary of your symptoms and medications to enable your doctor to make his best diagnosis. How true—but many people over look that point! This book is packed full of great advice and helpful hints!"

—Edie Adams
Actress/Model

"The need for optimism about aging is great; the optimism in this book is well founded."

—Jeanne E. Bader, Ph.D.
Gerontology,
Califonia State University, Long Beach

"This book is amazingly encyclopedic in scope and provides extremely valuable guidelines for just about everything in the lives of today's seniors/elders. It is an important addition to every household."

—Beverly Garland
Motion Picture and Television Star

"Whether designing your own future or helping someone you love, this book is essential for elders and caregivers alike. The wise choices we make today empower us with independence tomorrow."

—Jack Horak, Chair
California Commission on Aging

"My current lecture schedule calls for an average of 75 talks a year––most of them to Senior audiences. Overwhelmingly, they react enthusiastically to my central theme: How to make the BEST of the REST of your life. Your book is a perfect illustration of my main points and your authorities are impressive. Congratulations!"

—Art Linkletter
Television Personality/Author/Lecturer

Continued

"With this book, hope is no longer on the horizon. It is here now, alive and well! The door has opened and it's your turn to choose."
—Ed McMahon
Television Personality

"This text assists older Americans [in making] real choices for a life of independence."
—Joseph F. Prevratil,
President and CEO
Archstone Foundation

"[*The Wisdom To Choose*] provides a wealth of information that enables older adults to make informed choices in all aspects of their lives. [It is a] book that every older adult should have."
—The Rev. Charles Tindell, Chaplain
Minnesota Masonic Home
Bloomington, MN

"Dixon Arnett and Wende Chan provide an unusually comprehensive yet deep examination of the many elements that confront population aging. Not content to simply provide a listing of programs and services for older persons, they branch out to the 'wisdom' variables of spirituality, prevention and compassion. This book will be an important contribution to all who are aging."
—Fernando Torres-Gil, Ph.D., Director,
UCLA Center for Policy Research on Aging

"This book is a clear and simple roadmap to guide the elderly in our society. Use it as a reference and Arnett and Chan can be of great help in finding your way."
—Adam West
Actor/Author/Farmer

"This book serves as a great roadmap in helping us with positive choices. It shows us how to make the most of what we *can* do as we age, rather than thinking about the can'ts."
—Betty White
Actress/Author

About the Authors

Dixon Arnett served for thirty years in public office. His most recent assignment was as Director of the California Department of Aging, the largest state unit on aging in the nation. There, through California's 33 area agencies on aging, he administered the Older Americans Act and presided over the first major revision in the Older Californians Act since its inception. During his tenure he successfully pushed an initiative that resulted in the first funding increases in Older Californians Act services in almost a decade.

Previously, Arnett served in local, state and federal offices in posts that focused on health, social services and education. He served on the staff of the U.S. Senate, was Deputy Under Secretary of the U.S. Department of Health & Human Services and was a California State Assemblyman in the 1970s.

Wende Dawson Chan has been active in aging programs in San Francisco, spanning services from advocacy for nursing home residents to hospice care. She has been a caregiver to the end of life in her own home and for friends.

Chan has served three terms as a member of the federally-mandated Advisory Council to the San Francisco Commission on Aging and three years as an Ombudsman—part of the Older Americans Act that provides for a highly trained volunteer force to act as friends and advocates for residents in nursing homes.

Chan recently was elected Convener of the San Francisco Gray Panthers, an activist advocacy organization whose slogan is, "Youth and Age in Action." Her credentials include managing dental offices and serving on the Speakers' Bureau for the League of Women Voters.

Both Arnett and Chan have been project directors for "Community Outreach for Independent Living (COIL)," a California State-funded outreach effort to older and functionally-impaired adults. COIL reaches out through the use of community InfoVans and other means, so that seniors can make informed choices about lifestyle and social services.

THE WISDOM TO CHOOSE

THE WISDOM TO CHOOSE

A Comprehensive Guide
To Health and Independence For Elders

by
Dixon Arnett
and
Wende Dawson Chan

With a Foreword by
Jeanette Takamura
Assistant Secretary for Aging, 1997-2001
U.S. Department of Health and Human Services

The Wisdom To Choose
A Comprehensive Guide to Health and Independence for Elders

Copyright 2002 by Studio 4 Productions
Published by Studio 4 Productions
Post Office Box 280400
Northridge, CA 91328-0400
U.S.A.

Library of Congress Catalog Card Number: 2001-132907

ISBN: 1-882349-15-6

Editor: Bob Rowland

Book Design: Carey Christensen

Cover Design: Bob Aulicino

TABLE OF CONTENTS

APPENDIX A

FOREWORD

We are entering the 21st century with the gifts of health and longevity available to more and more Americans. What *The Wisdom To Choose* celebrates is the independence expressed by greater numbers of older persons in their daily lives.

Contrary to popular myths and stereotypes, most older Americans are in fact living independently and are actively involved in a spectrum of activities in their communities. Fewer are nursing home residents than ever before. Thanks to healthier lifestyles, public health, occupational safety, and other advances, a smaller proportion—6.5 percent fewer today than in 1982—are disabled.

There are many reasons why older Americans are likely to be living at home and in their communities. Study after study has confirmed the continuing support of family members and friends. Moreover, older Americans' longstanding preference for services to be provided in their homes or in community settings has been heard and is receiving increasing support from policy makers, funding agencies, and the private sector. And, in recent years, wonderful developments in technology have made it possible for health status monitoring and care to be provided right at home, instead of in doctors' offices or institutions.

Dixon Arnett and Wende Dawson Chan know well the fierce determination for independent living that most Americans share. They believe that the choices that we make determine the quality of our lives, however long or short our lives might be. Some choices may be better for certain persons than others. Nonetheless, each choice comes with its own set of consequences and its own advantages and benefits. Thus, as we each pursue quality in our own lives, we must ensure that we have the wisdom to choose in hand.

My friends and colleagues, Dixon and Wende, offer a guide to your choices. It is written for you, and you are strongly encouraged to engage your family and friends and caregivers in talking and thinking through your options. As you do so, you will be opening the door for them to also begin the process of acquiring knowledge, considering and thinking, and ultimately of having the wisdom to choose their own quality of life. But, never forget, you have the right to choose what will be best for you and your life.

May life be long and full of grace,
Jeanette C. Takamura
Assistant Secretary for Aging, 1997-2001
U.S. Department of Health and Human Services

INTRODUCTION:
OUR ELDERS, THEIR FAMILIES
AND CAREGIVERS

To Our Elders:
What Kind of Life Do You Want?

Choices! Consumer choices. Personal choices. Patient choices.

Choices to enhance spiritually and heighten your sense of yourself and your personal fulfillment and empowerment.

We are not "selling" anything here, other than the idea that you have choices in life that you may not know you have.

Throughout your life you have developed certain patterns, based on the energy of your spirit. This has to do with the very essence of who you are, what you think of yourself, and how you will live as an elder in your family or community. It has to do with how you "connect" with other people—how you make your ideas known to them, how you interact with them, and how you understand their preferences.

You will have the assistance of many when, and if, you want it. Of course, you can choose not to choose, if that's what you want—in which event, this book may inform without being of use to you. But even that is your choice.

What kind of life do you want? What kind of life have you led until now? What have been your surroundings? What are your thoughts about music, art, and reading? Are you a "people person," or do you prefer being alone (which doesn't necessarily mean "lonely")? These are among the choices you have made already, but we know that your choices are probably not one absolute preference over another. It's a mix of a composite lifestyle, and we hope you will listen to who you are, who you have been, and who you want to be.

This empowers you to know yourself so that your choices can be reflected in the way you live. In today's world, with extended life expectancies and new medical technologies bursting forth almost daily, you will have decades to craft a lifestyle that can free you from past constraints and let you live your own rediscovery.

According to a recent survey conducted by the Alliance for Aging Research, older Americans do not fear death as much as they fear developing Alzheimer's Disease or having to go into a nursing home. But, while Alzheimer's is a major catastrophe (although there is a full support system of services for patients and families), and while nursing homes can be debilitating, the vast majority of older Americans avoid Alzheimer's and nursing homes.

We contend that such avoidance—and the resulting independence and fullness of life—is something that each person can control, not completely, but in great measure. It seems to us that the fear of Alzheimer's and of nursing homes is, in fact, the fear of loss of control over one's own life.

The matter of self-appraisal is one that you should confront periodically. There is no one time for self-appraisal. It can be done as often as you wish. And, yes, you most certainly *can* change your mind. After all, we do that throughout our lives, as circumstances, some of which we may not control, take place.

The design of your own "game plan," based on your likes and dislikes, will provide a quality of life and a peace of mind that can benefit you directly and personally. If you seem forced to design a "game plan" for yourself that emphasizes accommodating others, be sure that you derive your own pleasure from such selflessness. Otherwise, you will stifle your own expression of yourself and risk becoming as dependent on others as if you were in an institution.

To Families and Caregivers: Useful Information

In this book, we lead you through essential information on health care (including major conditions affecting older Americans and the health programs for which older adults qualify) and the connection between mind and body. Throughout this guide, we emphasize the whole person, living in an environment conducive to independence of mind. We suggest pauses to contemplate re-framing of life, if that is a choice, "spiritual eldering," and making peace with death and dying.

We ask you to look around at your elders' environment (the things that surround them) and see what meaning they have. We suggest that you assess how your elders spend their time and what interests them. And, of course, we include a stop at the well of financial security, where you can evaluate your financial ability to do the things you want to do and be the person you want to be when you are elderly (which is perhaps not that far off).

We show you the path to community resources and social services from which you and your elders can choose. These services, most of which are free, are for your use, as well as theirs.

But what if there is a catastrophe? It can happen to anybody. A stroke or a severe fall, the onset of dementia or an accident from which it is hard to recover. All these, and others, may mean institutionalization. That may not be what you or your elders want, but, when it is needed, it's good that it's there. Does this mean that you lose all your choices in life? Certainly not! Our guide will explain some of those choices, too.

To Our Elders, Families and Caregivers Alike

Finally, there is a multitude of organizations-government, for-profit and non-profit—that can provide information at an instant. We'll guide you to them. They are valuable resources, and they will advocate for you.

Do we mean to picture some kind of nirvana? No. But we *do* mean to show you a map that will lead you through the continuum of living and, where appropriate, through assisted living and on to skilled nursing living, if that becomes necessary. Always, however, we intend to show that we all can live as independently as possible as long as possible.

According to a recent survey by the Department of Aging, in California alone, there are more than 67,000 volunteers helping to provide social services in the home and at senior centers at an in-kind value that exceeds the federal and state budgets for those same programs. These social services provide more independent living because the growing network of volunteers, caregivers, and government programs now reaches far more people. But you can choose them only if you know about them and can gain easy access to them.

In the very design of this book—with techniques of questionnaires and page format—we have devised a map for you to consult in making choices. Most importantly, we point out that you have choices you may not know you have.

Dixon Arnett   Wende Dawson Chan

YOUR BODY:
HEALTH AND LONG LIFE

The ABCs of Preventative Care

The human body is a complicated wonder of creation. The fact that all our parts seem to come together at the time of birth and, for the most part, function throughout life so that we have physical life support for our mental challenges and interactions with others, is truly a "wonderment."

But we cannot make the mistake of thinking that such "wonderment" is beyond us. Far more than we think, we *do* control our bodies, which, in turn, impacts our mental well-being. If we say to ourselves that the Creator of our bodies meant for us to be beyond our own wills, then that same Creator would not have given us a will of our own. But we *do* have a will, and we *do* have choice—especially about our bodies. But do we have the wisdom to choose?

In most societies, it is the older people who are supposed to have the wisdom of the years—the wisdom to teach and the wisdom to help others make decisions for either their own encouragement and benefit or for the overall good of a community. Therefore, one appeal to the older adults of our society is to have the "wisdom to choose"—for themselves and for the benefit of family and community.

The ABCs of preventative care, as technically complicated as our bodies may be, are as easy as the ABCs we learned in school as children. And, if those ABCs become habits, they give us a physical quality of life as surely as basic ABCs lead to language, articulation, and communication.

Simple reviews of the prevailing literature on prevention of almost every imaginable condition, ailment, or disease—regardless of a person's age—reveal common denominators that can prevent illness, or at least diminish it so that quality of life is not drastically impaired. While it is hard to establish a percentage—or even a range of percentages—of diminished quality of life, there are certainly plenty of data contained in major reports showing that choosing to be respectful of your body vastly diminishes your chances of experiencing debilitating illness and pain.

The following seminal documents focusing on prevention have been developed over two decades:

- *Healthy People: The Surgeon General's Report on Health Promotion and Disease Prevention*, 1979

- *Promoting Health/Preventing Disease: Objectives for the Nation*, 1980 (outlining 226 health objectives over 10 years)
- *Healthy People 2000: National Health Promotion and Disease Prevention Objectives*, 1991
- *Physical Activity and Health: A Report of the Surgeon General*, 1996
- *Healthy People 2010: Understanding and Improving Health*, 2000

These reports represent the work of thousands of experts and community leaders, writers, statisticians, researchers of medical literature and other resources, and advisors on leading health indicators. They also represent the work of planners, contributing authors, peer reviewers, senior reviewers, editors, editorial board members, and community resource leaders. They are composite works on diet and nutrition and fitness and exercise based on decades of research. Among health publications, they are undoubtedly the most often quoted resources in the United States today.

The following themes addressed in these publications are part of the selected specific sections added here as ABCs:

- diet and nutrition,
- exercise and fitness,
- early detection/intervention (testing and results),
- resources and choices, and
- patient advocacy (primarily for oneself).

Just realizing that you *do* control your health, that you *do* have choices about it, and that you *can* change and live your life to the fullest gives you a lease on a quality of life you would not have otherwise. A healthy nation starts with healthy individuals. Listed here are the 28 focus areas of *Healthy People 2010*; there are 467 specific objectives in the report, targeted at 2010, to amplify on the focus areas.

"Healthy People 2010" Focus Areas

1. Access to Quality Health Services
2. Arthritis, Osteoporosis and Chronic Back Conditions
3. Cancer
4. Chronic Kidney Disease
5. Diabetes
6. Disability and Secondary Conditions
7. Educational and Community-Based Programs
8. Environmental Health
9. Family Planning
10. Food Safety
11. Health Communication
12. Heart Disease and Stroke
13. HIV
14. Immunization and Infectious Diseases
15. Injury and Violence Prevention
16. Maternal, Infant and Child Health
17. Medical Product Safety
18. Mental Health and Mental Disorders
19. Nutrition and Overweight
20. Occupational Safety and Health
21. Oral Health

In terms of life expectancy, the United States has held its own and improved slightly over the past ten years. But there are trade-offs: people may smoke less, but they are more overweight. More older people now understand the need for exercise, yet because they are creatures of habit, it is hard for them to give up the high-fat diet they were raised on in favor of the low-fat, high-fiber diet that combats weight gain and a host of maladies.

It is also true that there is a growing movement toward patients being stronger advocates for themselves (some would argue to the chagrin of some health professionals). There is still a long way to go before older Americans understand that they have choices, even when the advice of physicians is sought. But, to a greater extent, there is more questioning, more "second opinions," and more counseling and reliance on health "professionals" in addition to doctors.

Part of that awareness is the growing sense that patients must be more aware of the medical tests being ordered and administered and what to expect from these tests. And there is a growing sense that detecting symptoms early will lead to early testing, which can lead to early treatment of even the most feared diseases.

Still, far too many older Americans ignore warning signs, maintain fatty diets, and avoid exercise, and then expect their physicians to be magicians who can cure ills that could have been prevented—if only the patient had made better choices in life. And now there is hard research data to prove it, lest there be doubt.

"The benefits of physical activity," says the 2000 Surgeon General's Report on *Physical Activity and Health*," have been extolled throughout western history, but it was not until the second half of this century [the 20th century] that scientific evidence supporting these beliefs began to accumulate."

Following *Healthy People 2000*, a similar team of government-sponsored researchers issued *The 1995 Dietary Guidelines for Americans*, which became the basis for revisions in the government's vaunted nutritional "recommended daily allowance" (RDA) and included "physical activity guidance to maintain and improve weight—30 minutes or more of moderate-intensity physical activity on all, or most, days of the week." Research shows conclusively that physical activity benefits physiological function with positive effects on the major systems of the body (musculoskeletal, cardiovascular, respiratory, and endocrine systems). The report goes on: "These changes are consistent with a number of health benefits, including a reduced risk of premature mortality and reduced risks of coronary heart disease, hypertension, colon cancer and diabetes mellitus... [and can reduce] depression and anxiety, improve mood and enhance ability to perform daily tasks throughout the life span."

Physical Activity and Health: A Report of the Surgeon General

The following conclusions are not restricted on the basis of age except as noted:

1. People of all ages, both male and female, benefit from regular physical activity.
2. Significant health benefits can be obtained by including a moderate amount of physical activity (e.g. 30 minutes of brisk walking or raking leaves, 15 minutes of running, or 45 minutes of playing volleyball) on most, if not all, days of the week...
3. ...people who can maintain a regular regimen of activity that is of longer duration or of more vigorous intensity are likely to derive greater benefit.
4. Physical activity reduces the risk of premature death in general and of coronary heart disease, hypertension, colon cancer and diabetes mellitus, in particular. Physical activity also improves mental health and is important for the health of muscles, bones and joints.
5. More than 60 percent of American adults are NOT regularly physically active. In fact, 25 percent of all adults are not active AT ALL!
[6. and 7. These conclusions relate to the decline in physical activity among younger people.]
8. More research on understanding and promoting physical activity [needs to be done], but... interventions to promote physical activity through...health care settings have been evaluated and found to be successful.

The President's Council on Physical Fitness and Sports, in a pamphlet entitled *Walking for Exercise and Pleasure*, points out how easy it is. "Walking," it says, "is the slower, surer way to fitness."

Almost everyone involved in the "aging network" has joked that his/her real job is to pick up where Ponce de Leon left off. He, of course, was the Spanish explorer who was steeped in the myth of the lost Fountain of Youth. Legend has it that if de Leon ever found the fountain, he didn't share his secret. Nor did he ever benefit directly, for he was buried in the 16th century.

Some say that the Fountain of Youth is within us; that is, there are chemicals that fight the effects of age. While researchers have identified chemicals that may help prevent disease, there is no magic elixir that arrests the aging process. Yet the body acts to counter certain "invasions" that can accelerate aging:

Antioxidants fight what are called "oxygen free radicals"—molecules that can be harmful to the energy-building cells in your body. Some of these "radicals" can come from an adverse environment such as smoke, radiation, and sunlight. The body battles these effects, mostly successfully, but as we age, the "radicals" can accumulate. Experts agree that the best way to assist your body in this battle is to eat fruits and vegetables that carry with them vitamins C and E and beta carotene, which is related to vitamin A. Depending on quality and absorption rates in your body, vitamin pills can help, but they are not as effective as whole fruits and vegetables, especially those that are fresh and not tainted with pesticides.

DNA contains and transmits your genes in every cell of your body. Routinely, every day, your DNA is "damaged" through normal use, and every day it is "repaired" naturally. But as we age, our bodies can fall behind on the "repairs," and the "damage" can build up. That's why there are some profit-makers who are eager to sell synthetic versions of DNA with the false promise that they will stop the aging process in its tracks. Their product is sold in pill form, which, when taken, dissolves into other substances and can't get to the cells to do any good. **Taking these pills does not stop the aging process!** The following table outlines the *normal* effects of the aging process.

Normal Physiological Changes of Aging

From *Aging in Good Health: A Complete, Essential Medical Guide for Older Men and Women and Their Families*
by Mark H. Beers, M.D. and Stephen K. Urice, Ph.D., J.D.
Reference/Pocket Books, New York, 1995

Organ	Age-Related Changes	Indicators
Brain	Blood flow decreases Chemical changes	Fainting can occur Confusion can occur
Eyes	Lens stiffens Retina less sensitive	A little blurring Difficulty seeing in dim light
Ears	Less able to hear	Difficulty in understanding

Continued

Mouth	Fewer taste buds	May lack, have bitter taste
Nose	Less able to smell	Many foods taste bland
Heart	Lowered pulse rate	Fainting may occur
	Lowered blood output	Sports activity fades
	Heart muscle stiffens	Heart failure may occur
	Response lowers	Less increase in heart rate
Lungs	Less air w/each breath	Exercise more difficult
	Less oxygen to blood	Hard breathing/high altitudes
Liver	Less blood flow and...	Medications reach higher levels in body,
	Less active enzymes longer	last longer
Kidneys	Less blood flow	Medications last longer
	Urine less dense	Dehydration can result
	Less salt excretion	May lead to kidney failure
Bladder	Wall muscles weaken	More difficult to urinate
	Less delay in urination	Can mean incontinence
Prostate	Enlarges	Urinary retention common
Skin	Underlying fat thins	Wrinkles occur, skin tears, hypothermia-cold sensitivity
Immune System	Fewer antibodies	Infections can occur and spread more quickly

Metabolism	Blood sugar levels rise	Probably none, but possible diabetes

DHEA is a substance said to boost the immune system and fight some kinds of cancer. Our bodies naturally contain DHEA sulfate, but the levels tend to decline as we age. You can buy substances labeled as DHEA that are said to supplement the body's supply, with the implication that it will retard the aging process; but there is no evidence—yet—that these substances are effective.

Note for women: DHEA is a precursor to hormones, and you may tend to give weight to DHEA as treatment. But remember that about 80% of substances labeled as DHEA, which are ingested orally, are "deactivated" by the liver, meaning that four-fifths of the value of the substance is passed through in your urine.

While products manufactured to mimic antioxidants, DNA and DHEA may do no harm, they do no good either in terms of retarding aging. Claims to the contrary are without foundation. Consider the warning given by the U.S. Administration on Aging on its web site (www.aoa.dhhs.gov/aoa/pages/agepages/lifextsn.html):

> "Currently no treatments, drugs, or pills are known to slow aging or extend life in humans. Check with a doctor before buying pills or anything else that promises to slow aging, extend life, or make a big change in the way you look or feel."

The key words in this warning are "…known to slow aging or extend life…". There is no Fountain of Youth, yet there are certain chemical or natural treatments that can make the quality of your life better, especially if there is some pain or discomfort to be dealt with.

According to the National Institute on Aging Information Center, there are plenty of ways we can help ourselves live long, healthy, and productive lives—ways that require little of us but common sense and decent habits. If your objective is to live a long life and stay healthy, then the Administration on Aging, along with the U.S. Surgeon General, has its own set of "Ten Tips For Healthy Aging" for you to consider—not unlike the advice given by the Surgeon General and *Healthy People 2010*. These rules, to the extent that you choose, can be your own "Declaration of Independence"—independent living and an independent lifestyle.

Ten Tips for Healthy Aging

1. Eat a balanced diet, including five helpings of fruits and vegetables a day.
2. Exercise regularly (check with a doctor before starting an exercise program).

Note!

Have you ever heard of an official government document advising you to "do things that make you happy" (see Tip #10)?

Well, there is at least one other: **The Declaration of Independence,** in which the founders say

3. Get regular health checkups.
4. Do NOT smoke (it's never too late to quit).
5. Practice safety habits at home to prevent falls and fractures; always wear your seat belt in a car.

> "that all men are endowed...with certain unalienable rights, that among these are life, liberty and the pursuit of happiness."
>
> Finding your own happiness, of course, means having your own choices.

6. Stay in contact with family and friends; stay active through work, play, and community.
7. Avoid overexposure to the sun and the cold.
8. If you drink, moderation is the key; when you drink, let someone else drive.
9. Keep personal and financial records in order to simplify budgeting and investing; plan long-term housing and money needs.
10. Keep a positive attitude toward life; do things that make you happy.

The Standards You Choose

All of us have been cajoled over the years to live a healthier lifestyle. Some of us have heeded the advice; some have ignored, or even scorned, it; and some have taken it, at least in part.

The purpose of this section is to give you choices—NOT to make you feel guilty. It is intended to give you a sense of confidence in yourself—NOT to make you a person measured against the standards of others, but ONLY the standards you choose.

The following set of questions demonstrates lifestyle habits which, if followed, avoid the most life-threatening illnesses and accidents.

- Do you regularly use a seat belt?
- Do you avoid "high-fat" foods?
- Do you choose a "high-fiber" diet?
- Do you attempt to lose weight (within reason)?
- Do you exercise regularly?
- Do you avoid exposure to the sun?
- Do you use sunscreen when in the sun?
- Do you make efforts to reduce stress in your life?
- Do you not smoke and avoid exposing yourself to second-hand smoke?
- Do you know how to conduct a self-examination for breast cancer (women) or prostate cancer (men)?

Answers to these questions invariably include qualifications and stories that are part of personal medical histories. For example, you may have smoked for years, but stopped recently.

As time marches on, there seem to be

Academicians, using a modern description of the steps of change, call it the "Trans-Theoretical Model:"

1. First, there is no contemplation of change, then...

constant reminders that changes in lifestyle will correct the "sins" of the past and prolong life. That may be so, but if those reminders make you feel guilty about the environment in which you grew up or advanced in your adult years, remember that your generation of seniors is the one that produced the very advances in medical technology that benefit all of us today. And, the environment of your younger years is part of the character you are today!

Thus, you can take

2. There is contemplation and a resolve to change (which can take a few minutes or several years), then...

3. There is the preparation of a change plan, then...

4. Action, over a 6-month time frame (the least stable period of change but during which there can be backup from family, friends, and support groups), then...

5. Maintenance of the action to change, after which...

6. There can be termination, or limiting, of the change or acceptance of, and even a comfort level with, the change.

pride in who you are and what you have done to bring renewed life to yourself as well as your children and grandchildren. At the same time, you can accept, if you wish, the suggestions of some who want you to live longer and more independently—if only you will CHOOSE to accept modest changes in your life.

But how do any of us change? Must we change overnight? Or can we be slower and more deliberate in making changes? What are the natural steps to bringing about change?

At the center of a decision, over time, to change one's lifestyle is a fundamental focus on self-interest. To be honest, change may not always be the result of a desire for perfect health or long life. But, for whatever reason(s), lifestyle changes that benefit health and long life can be made.

If you aspire to the long life that is being lived by greater numbers of people, the authors of *Living To 100* want to ask you a few questions. Your answers could mean you will live to be a centenarian (a person 100 years of age)—an exponentially growing segment of our aging population.

The principals of "The New England Centenarian Study," jointly conducted by the Harvard Medical School and Beth Israel Deaconess Medical Center, developed what they call a "Life Expectancy Calculator." Testing your "expectancy" is not a prediction of certainty. The questions result from studies of lifestyle risk factors and re-

Choosing to Change

There is the story of a man who, after a divorce, quit smoking because he knew that greater numbers of women whom he might date didn't like smoking, including second-hand smoke.

He might not have had the motives to quit that one finds in articles that discuss healthy habits—and it wasn't that he felt guilty about smoking for more than 20 years. Nevertheless, he quit for his own reasons.

Was he wrong? No! He cleared his lungs and started to live a healthier lifestyle.

flect the experience of the centenarians interviewed. The questions, and the reasons for them, featured in *Living To 100*, can be found on the Internet at www.beeson.org (click on "What Is Your Life Expectancy") or www.beeson.org/Livingto100/quiz.htm.

The web site automatically evaluates your answers and rates your life expectancy in years. Your test answers reflect your current lifestyle and should be instructive.

"The average person is born with a set of genes that would allow them to live to 85 years of age and maybe longer," says the Calculator's preamble. "People who take appropriate preventative steps may add as many as 10 quality years to that. People who fail to heed the messages of preventative medicine may subtract substantial years from their lives."

The "Living to 100"
Life Expectancy Calculator

These questions were asked of a large number of 100-year-olds in New England, based on lifestyle risk-factor studies. Their answers reflect their choices in life and imply that they lived to 100 because of the choices they made. (The factors used in weighting your answers and calculating your life expectancy are proprietary but generally described in Living To 100.)

The desired answer for each question ("Yes" or "No") depends on the reason for the question shown in parentheses. Your rating, under or over the average life expectancy of 85, depends largely on the lifestyle you have chosen for yourself.

Continued

Note: Non-italicized type in this section is from the Life Expectancy Calculator. Italicized type represents comments by the authors of this book.

- Do you smoke or chew tobacco, or are you around a lot of second-hand smoke? *(Cigarette smoke contains toxins that directly damage DNA and subsequently cause cancer.)*

- Do you eat more than a couple of hot dogs, slices of bacon, or a bologna sandwich a week? *(Some studies suggest that 90 percent of all human cancers are environmentally produced, 30 to 40 percent of these by diet.)*

- Do you cook your fish, poultry, or meat until it is charred? *(Charring food can change proteins and amino acids into carcinogens.)*

- Do you avoid butter, cream, sweets, and other saturated fats as well as fried food? *(High-protein diets, and the combination of a high-fat and protein diet, have been associated with increased risk of many types of cancer.)*

- Do you minimize meat in your diet, preferably making a point to eat fruits, vegetables, and bran? *(Diets that emphasize fruits and vegetables have been associated with significantly lower heart disease risk and better quality of life.)*

- Do you drink beer, wine, or liquor **in excess** (more than two drinks a day)? A standard drink is: one 12-ounce bottle of beer or wine cooler, one 5-ounce glass of wine, or 1.5 ounces of 80-proof distilled spirits. *(Excessive alcohol is toxic.)*

- Do you drink beer, wine, or liquor **in moderate amounts** (1-2 drinks a day)? A standard drink is: one 12-ounce bottle of beer or wine cooler, one 5-ounce glass of wine, or 1.5 ounces of distilled spirits. *(**Moderate** alcohol consumption has been associated with decreased heart disease risk; and is regarded by some studies to be beneficial.)*

- Do air pollution warnings occur where you live? *(A number of air pollutants are potent causes of cancer and contain oxidants that accelerate aging.)*

- Do you drink more than 16 ounces of coffee a day? Do you drink green tea, instead? *(Excessive coffee can both indicate and exacerbate stress.)*

- Do you take an aspirin a day? *(An 81 mg aspirin taken daily has been noted to significantly decrease the risk of heart disease. The benefit may be due to the anti-blood clotting effects of aspirin.)*

- Do you floss your teeth every day? *(Research shows that chronic gum disease leads to the release of inflammatory substances and bacteria into the blood stream that lead to heart disease.)*

- Do you have a bowel movement less than once every two days? *(Keeping gut transit time under 20 hours seems to decrease the incidence of colon cancer.)*

Continued

- Do you engage in risky (unprotected or promiscuous) sexual or drug-related behavior that increases your risk of contracting HIV or viruses that can cause cancer? *(Viruses such as HIV that are transmitted as a result of high-risk behavior not only cause AIDS but also various cancers, including lymphoma.)*

- Do you try to get a suntan? *(The association between sun exposure and accelerated aging is clear. The ultraviolet rays in sunlight directly damage DNA.)*

- Are there dangerous levels of radon in your house? *(Radon is a gas emitted from various types of rock, especially granite, that can accumulate to dangerous levels in people's homes. Toxic levels of radon in the home are equivalent to smoking two packs of cigarettes a day.)*

- I weigh ___ lbs. And my height is __ feet, __ inches. *(Being overweight is associated with inefficient energy production and an increased production of oxygen radicals within cells, leading to increased risk of various cancers and heart disease. Being obese [very overweight] multiplies that risk. The "Calculator" will automatically determine whether you are overweight and the relative degree to which you are overweight, if you are, based on published norms.)*

- Do you live near enough to other family members (other than your spouse and dependent children) that you can drop by spontaneously? *(Extended fam-*

ily cohesiveness and frequent contact is a notable feature of centenarian families.)

- Which statement is applicable to you? "Stress eats away at me; I can't seem to shake it off," or, "I can shed stress" [this might be accomplished by praying, exercising, meditating, being able to respond to humor, or by other means]. *(Centenarians shed emotional stress exceptionally well.)*

- Does more than one member of your immediate family (parents and siblings) have diabetes? *(Diabetes causes excessive exposure to glucose and, when uncontrolled, results in the onset of age-related problems.)*

- Did both your parents die before age 75 years of non-accidental causes? Or did they both (or one of them if the other died before age 75) require assistance by the time they reached age 75? *(Genetics plays a significant role in the ability to achieve extreme old age.)*

- Did more than one of the following relatives in your family live to at least 90 years in excellent health: parents, aunts/uncles, or grandparents? *(If you have significant extreme longevity in your family, this will help significantly in your ability to achieve old age in good health.)*

- Are you a couch potato? Do you exercise 20 minutes a day or more? *(Exercise leads to more effi-*

Continued

cient energy production and a lower production of age-accelerating free radicals in our cells. Exercise has been linked to lower rates of breast and prostate cancer. NOTE: Only 36 percent of male baby boomers, and only 35 percent of female baby boomers, exercise regularly.)

- Do you take vitamin E (800IU) and selenium (100-200 mcgm) every day? *(Vitamin E is thus far the best scientifically proven anti-oxidant available, either in the diet or as a dietary supplement; selenium appears to have dramatic effects in preventing cancer.)*

Note: After answering the above questions on the web site, click on the CALCULATE YOUR LIFE EXPECTANCY button for calculation results.

Relevant links to the Centenarian Study web site are: The Alliance for Aging Research, The Paul Beeson Physician Faculty, Scholars in Aging Research Program, Shape-Up America!, the American Heart Association, the American Lung Association, and PBS's *Stealing Time*.

Common Sense

Caregiving

The term *caregiver* connotes love and attention, a voluntary giving of one's self to another. Few goals in life could be loftier. But few goals have as much chance to go wrong, perhaps even adding to feelings of loneliness born of misunderstanding.

There are essentially two roles in caregiving: (1) the individual as his/her own best caregiver; and (2) the individual as the receiver of caregiving. To be successful, both must involve giving and understanding.

There is a strong, growing movement to empower you, the older adult and the elderly, first and foremost. Your family members and friends need to learn how unique you are as an elder and that the life you have led represents who you are and the choices you are likely to make. They ought to understand that you know, far better than anyone else, the best choices for you.

You, in fact, are your own best caregiver; that is, first you must care for yourself in a loving and attentive manner, accepting responsibility for making choices for yourself and accepting the consequences of those choices. Give yourself life and express yourself, and you will be able to accept the help of others as you need it. Give yourself respect, and you will find others more likely to respect your wishes. Give yourself love and attention, and others will respond in kind. Honor your mind and body, and they will serve you well—certainly better than if you abuse them. In short, empower yourself so that your life will lift the lives of others.

Caregiving comes in many forms, from family to volunteers paid and unpaid, at home and in care facilities. The universal creed should be The Golden Rule: *"Do Unto Others as You Would Have Them Do Unto You."* (See page 85 et. seq. for caregiver referral resources.)

Charles Tindell, Chaplain of the Minnesota Masonic Home, a nursing and assisted living facility in a Minneapolis suburb, has written a veritable tribute to "his" residents in a book entitled, *Seeing Beyond The Wrinkles:*

Stories of Ageless Courage, Humor, and Faith (Studio 4 Productions, Northridge, CA, 1998).

Rather than focusing on the "hard" decisions younger generations have to make about elderly "Mom" and "Dad," Tindell looks at the lives and characters of the elderly who are in care facilities and concludes, in story after story, that there is a resiliency and verve

> ### Look for...
>
> *The Caregiver Pocket Reference*
> Adult Care Services, Inc.
> 844 Sunset Avenue
> Prescott, AZ 86305
> 520-445-6633
> May, 2000; $7.50

in those he writes about that gives meaning to life.

In his book, he gives us glimpses of character in stories of professional lives and accomplishments—from sea captains to frontier housewives, from depression-era newspaper boys to soldiers who fought the wars that preserved the same nation that nurtures their offspring.

Tindell shares the pathos and the humor, and often he shows us the resident who has taught himself how to make peace with dying and, thereby, teaches others even as he dies. These are *not* the stories of people who are warehoused, transfixed on the seemingly unchanging picture and monotone sound of a television set. No! These are the stories of people who are part of their lives, interacting with others and welcoming their friends and families as visitors to their home. Tindell sees the elderly as empowered, if they want to be. He sees them being respected as they respect themselves.

Now, contrast Tindell's view with stories describing the obvious anguish of sons and daughters who make a decision to admit an elderly parent into a nursing home. They may believe with every emotion in them that this is the beginning of the end; that their parent will never again be a part of their lives, except on periodic visits during which there will be fewer and fewer things to talk about because, of course, the assumption is that the parent will no longer have a life.

In Tindell's view, the elderly take care of themselves by using the services of others, by making reasonable demands on those who are providing services, and by not being afraid or too timid to ask. This contrasts with the depiction of the elderly as people to be pitied because they can't care for themselves any longer. For Tindell, the elderly are a source of wisdom (see also "Spiritual Eldering,"® page 104) and teaching through their stories and choices, not useless people to be put away in rooms, rarely to be heard from again.

In fact, you may have something to teach. Consider the experience of a 5th grade teacher near San Francisco who brought her class to visit a nursing home. There she found the sea captain who had sailed the last three-masted schooner around Cape Horn through billowing storms. He fascinated the children with his stories and gave them an experience they will remember for a lifetime.

Tindell, who has now published a sequel, represents a growing trend toward empowerment and away from patronizing attitudes toward the elderly. His version of caregiving is a partnership—a partnership in which the elderly resident in an institution, for example, is the boss.

In his view, caregiving is a partnership in which choices are to be made, if at all possible, by the resident—not the nurse or the doctor (except in emergencies) or the administration, which may be focused on "convenience" and the bottom line.

Thus, to be your own best caregiver, you must become knowledgeable about the choices you have, in or out of an institution, and about the services that are available, what they cost, and whether or not you have to pay for them. Invariably, there may be reasonable limits on your choices, but having those choices contrasts with the fact that many people don't believe they have a choice at all.

The caregivers who assist you do exactly that—assist. They do not command or order. No more "there, there, dear-y" on the part of the nurse, no more visits cut short by the doctor before you get a chance to finish your questions, and no more nutritionists who won't let you have a candy bar on your 100th birthday.

Whether you are caregiving for yourself or someone else, you may wonder, *What constitutes caregiving?* For a start, look again at the Table of Contents of this book. Using the contents as a checklist, where are you on the caregiving front? Are your money and legal matters organized? Do you need insurance? Do you have the money for the retirement you plan? What about your health and keeping well? Are you able to keep your body and mind together?

Have you assessed your own spirituality (aside, but not necessarily separate, from organized religion)? What about the environment in which you live? Do you have interests and activities that occupy you, including family and friends? Do you know what resources are available to you, from entertainment to transportation? Can you live independently, or do you need help with what is called "assisted daily living (ADLs—eating, dressing, bathroom functions)"? What organizations can you call on to assist you with everything from publications and information to advocating on your behalf? Are you prepared for emergencies, from the need for calling 911 to long-term illness? Do you have a quality of life that prepares you for the quality of dying and death?

These are all questions for you, but they are also questions for your caregiver(s). They should know *your* answers to these questions, too, so that if there are others helping you, then they will know your preferences. For good caregiving to be a fact, you and your caregiver must communicate often.

If you have a caregiver, you must think about him/her and try to understand the demands you make. Even national leaders are now beginning to pay attention to the very real costs of caregiving to those family members and friends who provide for others. There is renewed consideration of a tax credit for caregivers, and there is the start of congressional consideration of including caregiving as an amendment to the Family Leave Act.

Yet, caregiving, while being genteel, also can be smothering and patronizing, even condescending. Recently, several best-selling books purport to render caregivers advice (even providing checklists). But the "readers" are those who provide help to people who seem, according to the authors, to be virtually helpless. In this sense, the books may be well-meaning, but they are patronizing, making the assumption that most elderly people are without thought or personal preferences and have no choices.

It's as though the elderly, by definition, reach a time when physical needs render them without mental capacity, no personal history, no lifelong expressions. Granted that a certain number of the elderly in nursing homes are rendered helpless and totally dependent on others due to severe debilitating or terminal illness. But the *majority* retain their individual identities and can fully communicate their wishes.

To put you in touch with your feelings about caregiving, authors Barbara Silverstone and Helen Kandel Hyman have listed a set of emotional issues on caregiving in their book, *You and Your Aging Parent*. Their book, published in 1998, includes a test for the receiver of caregiving.

Where are you on these issues?

Facing Up to Feelings

From *You and Your Aging Parent*, by Barbara Silverstone and
Helen Kandel Hyman, Consumers Union,
Ed. © 1976, 1982; Printed in 1978, 1982

- The emotional **Tug of War:** Conflicts of love and annoyance or where one loves more than the other.
- **Love, Compassion, Respect, Tenderness, Sadness**: A progression of feelings which parents have for children when they are young and which children may return in kind toward their parents

---

when they are old. Some of these feelings may
exist apart from the others.

- **Indifference**: If these feelings exist apart, then it is
  possible to feel respect but not love or affection
  or even friendship. Lack of feeling may turn into
  remorse, but there still may be feelings of responsibility.
- **Love May Not Be Enough**: Love and affection can
  be liabilities if there is too much dependency on
  the person loved.
- **Fear and Anxiety**: Some live in fear that they will
  not live up to expectations.
- **Anger and Hostility**: Feelings over events or
  behaviors of the past can be as discomforting as
  tenderness can be comforting; it is important to
  learn from anger and avoid hostility.
- **Sexuality**: On this subject there needs to be adult
  respect by, and for, everyone.
- **Shame**: The feeling you are not doing enough.
- **Reactions to Aging**: Can you accept old age? Do
  you like people who are aging? Can you accept a
  different role? Are you overburdened?
- **Guilt**: Which can lead to resentment, which can
  lead to more guilt.

Taking Care of Yourself

Knowing who you are (your self-identity) is not a
simple task; it is a lifelong pursuit.

Throughout life, people construct a sense of identity and a system of beliefs about who they are and how
they feel. The first identification of a personal self in the

greater world may impact patterns of life in both mind and body. Each person is also born with an innate sense of what he or she can be and what he or she wants to do. The strength of this internal trajectory out into the world drives curiosity and enthusiasm.

When all works well, these "life forces" within are nourished and renewed by the patterns of living and skills each chooses to practice regularly. When things "fall apart" or there are challenges of overwhelming change around or within, the individual sense of indentity, belief system, the very body and soul, become vulnerable. In this shaky state it is hard to know what to do.

The regaining of a vital presence within yourself, and a vital connectedness beyond yourself, becomes necessary. But how is this renewal accomplished? One way is to engage in the following cycle of thought and action.

- Take inventory: what is left? What does work now? What has worked in the past? Conversely, what doesn't work? Are there things that need to be discarded?
- Seek support: These may be comfortable habits and old friends, which help renew the parts that do work.
- Discover new information: This includes understanding more about your situation, learning new skills, and consulting people more expert than yourself.
- Imagine, visualize, and plan: Imagine all the possibilities, visualize the ones that might work for you, and plan to accomplish change.

- Strengthen and rebuild: Put your plan into action.
- Test your new habits: This includes testing your own mastery of your plan of action and building immunities in both mind and body, being mindful of vulnerability in the future.
- Reflect and embrace: Allow yourself time and space to celebrate your success and feel the renewed sense of health and balance.

Diet and Nutrition

Balance and health at any age come from the choices each of us makes.

A 92-year-old watched his home health aide prepare his medicine, all the while eating a soft candy bar:

"That's really not good for you," she said. "It's just sugar and no nutrition."

"But, my dear," he said, "I am 92. How much will this candy bar affect the time I have left? I'll eat what I want to eat. It's too late for me to reform."

"Well, you have a point," she admitted. "But what quality of life do you want for the time you have left? Eating junk can upset your regularity and make you feel miserable. That won't make your days very happy ones."

"I guess you have a point, too," the man said. "But all you health people make it seem like I can only be healthy if I eat nothing but tofu, broccoli, and rhubarb— none of which I like. I want to enjoy what I eat, even if I don't have the teeth to bite down on a steak anymore."

"It's a compromise," she agreed. "Balance. That's the key. Of course, you can eat the things you like—even that candy bar, if you insist. That's your choice. And your choices come first. I'm just saying that your body will give you messages about what it needs. And you should pay attention."

"Well, you young whippersnappers seem to have all the answers," the man shot back, "but I didn't get to be 92 by not paying attention to what goes on around me and living my life pretty well."

"Just my point," she said. "You've made choices all your life—some good with great results, some bad with consequences. Nutrition is no different, whether you're 92 or 12!"

Food Facts for Older Americans

"According to a nationwide survey of doctors and nurses, a quarter of older Americans are malnourished. Many are not eating the foods they need to preserve their health and prevent a range of degenerative diseases which have come to be associated with aging, but which, in many cases, can be avoided by simple, low-cost changes in what we eat, and how we eat it."

– "Elder Action: Action Ideas for Older Persons and Their Families," U.S. Administration on Aging Fact Sheet, 1/22/00. Web site: www.aoa.dhhs.gov/aoa/eldractn/foodfact.html

---

*   *   *   *   *

Would it surprise you to know that most Americans were much healthier in terms of what they ate and their weight a hundred years ago? They consumed more calories, but they weighed less. The difference was diet and exercise. They didn't have the processed foods we have today, and they ate the vegetables they raised—not canned or frozen. Yes, they ate meat (and the fat of the meat), but they worked off their calories through the physical activity of agricultural and industrial jobs and household chores. Today, we don't get that kind of physical activity unless we make it a point to.

Nutritionists rightly suggest diets that include fiber—whole grains, cereals, beans, peas, lentils—and fruits. Fibers give you the feeling of being full because they absorb water and don't have many calories. One hundred years ago, Americans had twice as much fiber in their diet as they do today. Besides, fibers cleanse the intestinal tract, which prevents constipation, which, in turn, can be a factor in an hiatal hernia, hemorrhoids, and varicose veins. Even our 92-year-old would want to avoid these consequences, perhaps even more than those who are younger.

Conversely, Americans today are overweight on the average, primarily because we eat 30 percent more fat than our counterparts a century ago, without doing the exercise that burns off caloric fat. Researchers debate the level of fat that should be in our diet, but there seems to be agreement on somewhere between 10 and 30 percent (remember that cutting off the fat from meat doesn't eliminate the cholesterol [build-up of fatty substances] in the lean). If you are a heart patient, you have been instructed to cut back on fat intake, a change that can arrest, even reverse, arteriosclerosis.

The following warning is from the Administration on Aging:

> "Current research has found that a diet high in fat contributes to the incidence of late onset diabetes, atherosclerosis (which is a major cause of heart disease and strokes) and cancers of the colon and reproductive organs in both men and women."

Warnings such as this are not new, of course, but there is reason to believe that when we are younger, we ignore similar warnings about safety and avoiding risks in favor of adventure. But now our population is growing older—and wiser—so warnings that were disregarded make more sense to us because we want to live longer and live a quality of life our parents and grandparents only dreamed of (but also made possible for us).

Multiple studies demonstrate that the major diseases afflicting older Americans can be diminished or eliminated by changes in diet and exercise. Results in reversing arteriosclerosis have been dramatic, but read this, also from the Administration on Aging:

> "Researchers have found that populations that omit meat and dairy products from their diets, or use them sparingly, and eat large amounts of fruits, vegetables, nuts, seeds and starches such as rice, potatoes and cereal grains have a 40% lower incidence of cancer..."

These fiberous foods are high in vitamins C, E, and B complex, beta carotene, and folate, all of which help to reduce "free radicals" (molecules, often from smoking, that attack energy-building cells) in your body that can cause cell damage and lead to cancer. In addition to

vitamins, fiberous foods contain cancer-fighting ingredients called phytochemicals (groupings of body chemicals) that boost the synthesis of anti-cancer enzymes.
These enzymes actually fight to detoxify carcinogens.
This is why researchers report that fiber in the diet reduces the risk of cancers.

A word of advice, however—you can't go out and
gorge on junk food and then take vitamin pills, ratio-
nalizing that you have reduced your risk of cancer. The
vitamins don't contain the cancer-fighting phytochemicals; they are only in the fibers themselves. Vitamin pills
(supplements) can assist your diet significantly, but they
are not a substitute for natural vitamins in fibers; nor
are they antidotes for indulgence in foods that have no
redeeming vitamin value.

Where are the phytochemicals found? We all know
that former President George H.W. Bush didn't like his
broccoli, but that's one place where cancer-fighting
phytochemicals are found. They are also present in cau-
liflower, brussel sprouts, turnips, kale, and cabbage.
Tomatoes, onions, garlic, and soybeans are also part of
the anti-cancer army, as well as fruits like strawberries,
grapes, and raspberries. Former President Bush must
have found dietary friends in some of these other fibers, even if he didn't like broccoli.

Many of these same fibers are also important in fight-
ing osteoporosis, or bone loss due to loss of calcium.
They are a source of calcium, which is more readily ab-
sorbable than calcium found in dairy products. This
makes it important for women at risk for osteoporosis,
who are middle-aged or older, to enlist a fiber-strong
diet as an ally in preventing heart disease, cancer, and

osteoporosis. Estrogen/Progesterone therapy can help, but it is not appropriate for all women, whereas a higher-fiber, lower-fat diet is.

It should be noted that a new study by the Harvard School of Public Health has set aside previous notions that consumption of calcium increases the risk of developing kidney stones. In fact, the re-

---

Don't Drink Your Life Away

From Administration on Aging Elder Action: *Food Facts for Older Americans*, January 22, 2000.

"Researchers at Brigham and Women's Hospital in Boston and Harvard University found that people who consume more than two alcoholic drinks per day cancel out the benefits of eating large amounts of fruits and vegetables, and...are at higher risk of developing precancerous polyps in the colon..."

---

verse is true. In results from a study of more than 45,000 men, those with a higher-fiber diet, including calcium, had a one-third *less* risk of kidney stones. The same study said that those with the highest consumption of potassium, also found in a higher-fiber diet, had half the risk of developing kidney stones.

What's more, a higher-fiber diet is usually less expensive (depending on your cost of living) than fats, salty foods, and a diet that contains virtually no vitamins. Usually, a tasty salad and a piece of fruit will cost far less than a hot dog and a bag of potato chips of the same weight.

"You are what you eat." So goes the age-old expression. But it's not just an expression if it means that you can reduce the risk of disease, lose weight, boost your energy level, and look and feel your best by balancing your diet to rely less on fats, salts, and sugars while relying more on fiber, vitamins, and exercise.

Also, a word of consumer advice: vitamin supplements sold today, either over-the-counter or through direct sales, cover a span of value from nil to vital. Often, different supplements appear to contain the same ingredients, so consumers opt for cheaper brands. Sometimes, however, the cheaper brands do little or no good, even though they sound good. The difference is absorption in the body. If some vitamin supplements pass through your body quickly, then the supplement does little good. But, coupled with a higher-fiber diet, the supplement should be able to be absorbed so that it can provide you with the nutrients it contains. Don't hesitate to ask the advice of a physician or pharmacist before shopping for vitamins.

For More Information...

Food Guide Pyramid: A Guide to Daily Food Choices
Human Nutrition Information Service
U.S. Department of Agriculture, August 1992
Home and Garden Bulletin No. 252

Barnard, Neal, M.D., *Food for Life*, Harmony Books, 1993.

Ornish, Dean, M.D., *Dr. Dean Ornish's Program For Reversing Heart Disease*, Ballentine Books, 1991.

Doctor Dialogue

According to a cross-sectional study based on 1993 data published in the December 22/29, 1999 issue of the *Journal of the American Medical Association* (JAMA), 10 out of 11 doctor-patient office visits fail to meet the standards of communication that are determined by the medical profession itself. These are standards doctors themselves have determined are necessary for informed decision-making by patients.

But before finger-pointing begins, stop to think: **Are you doing your part to help your doctor help you?!** When we go to a physician, we often believe that, because the doctor has a medical degree, and because he or she wears those "badges" (a white smock and a stethoscope) that suggest status, we have no obligation to inform the doctor completely about ourselves.

Many patients think that doctors are magic "fix-it" men and women whose superior knowledge is a panacea. But common sense should dictate that physicians are human, like the rest of us. They can help you, yes. But you can improve their performance (and your health) simply by providing them with pertinent, timely information.

Patient-doctor dialogue is *not* just a matter of telling the doctor where you hurt. **It means telling the doctor as**

> "Primary care physician visits lasted a mean of 16.5 minutes... visits with surgeons lasted a mean of 13.6 minutes."
>
> –"Decision Making in Outpatient Practice," *Journal of the American Medical Association* (JAMA),vol. 282, no. 24, Dec. 22/29, 1999, p. 2317.

much as you can about your condition or pain and providing him or her with a full background of your medical history. It is also about being prepared to ask the doctor questions.

Similarly, physicians who voluntarily don white smocks and visible medical paraphernalia are advertising to patients that they possess training and knowledge that patients don't have, and that they can assist in curing ills, from minor to life-threatening. It is about as serious a profession as a person can choose.

Thus, licensing of physicians was started in the United States in the post-Civil War period. Initially, licensure was at the insistence of the medical profession itself—consistent with the Hippocratic Oath (requiring, in the first instance, that a physician "...shall do no harm...") and high professional standards.

Over time each state established its own medical licensing board, but as the nation became more litigious on behalf of consumers, these boards became major sources for information on, and discipline of, physicians who did not meet the standards of their licensure.

Recent annual data shows an average of complaints against 9 percent of physicians but investigations were warranted on only 5 percent and actual discipline on just under 2 percent. Put another way, over 90 percent will never receive even a complaint.

What Kind of a Patient Are You?

Here are some questions to answer about yourself. This is intended to be a self-assessment:

- Are you someone who keeps a copy of your own medical records? Can you describe your physical condition? Any persistent conditions? Do you know about the conditions of your immediate family?
- Do you maintain a list of the prescription drugs you are taking? (Be sure to include the name of the prescribing doctor and his or her phone number.)
- Do you have a list of over-the-counter drugs, vitamins, and supplements you take regularly? Do you carry a copy of the list?
- Do you exercise regularly? What kinds of exercise? How often? Do you know your height and weight?
- What are your eating habits? Can you describe them to your physician if he or she asks?
- Do you get appropriate physical examinations regularly? How often? What kinds of physicals? Modest or extensive?
- When you make an appointment with your physician because of some matter that is troubling you, do you write down your symptoms?
- Do you write down questions to ask?
- Do you ask about tests your physician wants to order?
- Do you ask for written instructions from your doctor?
- In short, are you ready to "partner" with your doctor?

What Kind of a Physician Are You?

Here are some self-assessment questions for physicians:

- How do you allocate your time? Are you a crisis doctor, or do you set aside enough time to do all you must do in an office visit? Or when discussing surgery? Do you allow extra time for patients and their families when you know the situation is serious? Life-threatening?
- Do you *initiate* communication with your patients? Do you ask them to prepare for the visit? In the course of the office visit, do you elicit discussion of not only symptoms but also medical history, medication management habits, and lifestyle habits? Do you take the time to ensure that your patient understands your questions? Do you take the time to follow up with the patient if you do not understand the answers, particularly if there are language difficulties?
- Are you as clear as you can be with your patients about diagnosis? Treatments and options? Remedies and options? Choices? Pros, cons, uncertainties?
- Do you make sure your patient understands what you have said before the patient leaves? Do you provide written instructions to your patients?
- Do you tell your patients that they have choices they should make?
- Do you wait for your patients to respond? In short, are you ready to "partner" with your patients?

But, because of their status, doctors *do* have a vital responsibility to initiate effective communication with their patients. In rare and extreme cases, when lack of communication is evident, the doctor may be guilty, literally, of "gross negligence."

For example, in most cases, if a physician prescribes a serious painkilling drug without ever seeing or evaluating the patient, that is considered "gross negligence." That sounds like common sense, yet there are patients who ask, and doctors who respond, with little thought given to possible consequences.

According to the JAMA-published survey, the average visit with a primary care physician lasts 16.5 minutes—and with a surgeon it lasts 13.6 minutes. That means, by definition, of course, that many of these visits are shorter.

Let's assume you have 16.5 minutes for a visit with your primary care physician to present him or her with a new illness or pain. Let's also assume that the doctor has your medical records and has at least glanced at them. During your brief visit, the doctor must:

- Try to put you at ease by being pleasant (bedside manner),
- Diagnose your illness, often by examination,
- Identify possible treatments, if not remedies,
- Make you, the patient, a "partner" by discussing your role as a patient in making a decision (particularly if the illness or pain is serious and requires choices with consequences),
- Discuss the clinical nature of your decision,
- Provide you with alternatives and their pros, cons, and uncertainties,

- Explore with you your preferences and try to assess whether you understand what has been said, and
- Finally, be as reassuring as possible as you leave.

All those tasks must be completed, but they don't have to be done in one visit, unless there is a crisis. If more than one visit is necessary, from your point of view because you are troubled or you have more unanswered questions (which is normal), then schedule another visit. Even the best communication may require more conversation.

Actually, the same JAMA-published study gave physicians decent marks (71 percent) in communicating diagnoses and treatments, but **only 1.5 percent of the doctors took the time to assess whether their patients understood.**

Only 5.9 percent of the doctors even told their patients that they had a role in the process at all. And alternative treatments were discussed only 11.3 percent of the time. The study's conclusions were based on 1,057 patient visits to 124 different doctors (59 were primary care physicians, and 65 were general and orthopedic surgeons).

By any measure, this is a dismal record for both doctors and patients.

Do you know that you may bring a family member or companion with you on your visit to your doctor?

If you consent, someone else being with you is okay within the doctor-patient relationship; it does not violate confidentiality.

Lack of time is not an excuse; neither is lack of preparation. Perhaps we expect too much of our physicians, but, by the same token, physicians too often take their patients for granted or consider them as part of an assembly line.

For example, two patients went to different doctors on the same day. One patient went with a list of five questions; the doctor answered only two and left saying he had other patients with greater urgencies. The other patient had five written questions as well. When the doctor saw that answering the questions would take time, he asked if he could be excused to tend to a patient fresh from surgery. He said that he would return so that both he and the patient could take the time required. The patient agreed. The doctor returned and spent 45 minutes answering those questions. Which one of those doctors would *you* have chosen to be your physician?

What does the JAMA-published study show? Certainly, the study, based on audiotapes, shows that doctor "dialogue" is missing in most cases. It also shows that when doctors don't initiate a "partnership" with their patients, the vast majority of those patients don't initiate communication either.

Both doctors and patients can take the time to be prepared for the average 16.5-minute visit. Doctors can read medical records; patients can list symptoms and medications being taken and make a note of the questions they want to ask. In fact, if it is convenient, leave your written questions at the doctor's office, or fax or e-mail them in advance of your scheduled visit.

What You Can Do to "Partner" with Your Doctor

1. Keep in touch with your primary care physician. As you consult with specialists, inquire to be sure that your primary care doctor and the specialists share information about you.

2. Keep copies of your medical records. Under the laws of all states, those records belong to you! Keep records of prescriptions, over-the-counter drugs, vitamins, and supplements you take (and carry a copy with you) and be prepared to tell any inquiring medical professional what you are taking and why. It's on the bottle!

3. Prepare for your appointment with your doctor by writing down your symptoms and your questions. Don't expect your doctor to anticipate your questions.

4. Ask if there are videotapes, articles, pamphlets, or Internet sites you can review before your visit.

5. Be totally open about your lifestyle habits and personal beliefs that might, in any way, have an effect on your treatment. Write them down; give them to your doctor. Your talks with your doctor are private and privileged.

6. If you need another appointment to satisfy your questions as a patient, make one, and explain why!

Be sure you understand the tests your physician wants you to take. Even a simple blood test may have

aspects to it that you should know. The questions you
should ask are simple, but the answers can be quite serious, depending on the type of illness your physician
suspects. Give careful consideration to the following
questions:

- What does your doctor expect the test to reveal? Or what does he or she think might be
  learned by the test? Are there certain possible
  diagnoses your doctor wants to rule out?
- Are there any risks in taking the test? (There
  is little risk to you in drawing your blood,
  but there may be discomfort or pain in more
  invasive tests.)
- What will happen if you do not consent to
  the test? How will your condition, illness, or
  pain progress without the test?
- How long will it take to learn the results of
  the test?
- What is the rate of "false positives" or "false
  negatives" in the test your doctor wants you
  to take? How will your doctor take these factors into account?

Clearly the more serious the possible diagnosis, the
more vital these issues are. Do not take the prospect of
tests for granted. You have a right to know the answers
to the questions listed above (and others you may have).
Always ask!

NOTE: In most states it is illegal for a physician to
refer you to a laboratory in which he or she owns a financial interest. It is considered a conflict of interest,
simply because of the appearance, if not the fact, of ordering unnecessary tests on which the physician doing

the ordering is making money. As noted, every state has a medical board that licenses and regulates physicians. Most of these boards have a toll-free telephone number for you to call when you need to know the status (public record) of the doctor in whom you are entrusting your care.

Exercise and Fitness

"I'm no Arnold Schwarzenegger!"—"I'm no Jane Fonda!"

Well, you don't have to be. You don't have to be the former chairman of the California Governor's Council on Physical Fitness and Sports, or the CEO of your own chain of fitness salons and TV aerobic shows. You don't even have to be a movie star in the ultra-thin world of Hollywood to get into your own regular exercise regimen.

In fact, if you do not now have a regular exercise program, and you start right

> ### *When You Do Not Exercise...*
>
> - ...fat displaces muscle,
> - ...muscles become smaller and weaker (known as atrophy),
> - ...you gain weight more easily because fat burns less calories than muscle, and
> - ...added body weight puts more stress on your heart, lungs and on the weight-bearing joints of your hips, knees, and ankles.
>
> From *Fitness Facts for Older Americans*, U.S. Administration on Aging, January 22, 2000: www.aoa.dhhs.gov/aoa/eldractn/fitfact.html

out trying to be Schwarzenegger or Fonda, you could seriously hurt yourself. People like Schwarzenegger and Fonda have spent their entire lives building their bodies, so don't try to duplicate their acumen in record time.

But using Schwarzenegger or Fonda as a foil for lack of exercise is a poor excuse. They certainly don't intend themselves to be a foil for anyone's lack of motivation. Only about one-third of all Americans 45 and older exercise regularly. That includes everyone from famous fitness experts to average men and women who start, perhaps, with stretching exercises or swimming and go on to serious aerobics.

Exercise is anything you do that involves "resistance" or "aerobics"—anything that you keep doing with slight increases in degree so that you are always challenging yourself. For example, if you are not now exercising at all, you might start with stretching exercises and brisk walks for about 20 minutes a day. In time, you can increase the stretching to swimming a lap or two at your community pool, if you have one, or mild calisthenics. Later, you can swim several laps, walk a mile slightly uphill, or do floor calisthenics that will strengthen your "abs" (abdominal muscles).

As you progress with regular exercise, the human body can repair itself, particularly the muscloskeletal (muscles and bones) system and the cardiovascular-pulmonary system (lungs and heart, including the miles of veins, arteries, and capillaries in our bodies). For example, exercises that strengthen the muscles in the back along the spinal column will help take the weight of standing and bending and thus allow joints and discs in the column to repair in time.

Conversely, lack of exercise puts pressure on bones to carry your weight without rebuilding them, which makes them more brittle (osteoporosis). It becomes more difficult to climb stairs, get out of a chair, or maintain balance. We are more prone to falls. But regular exercise can help prevent these shortfalls. You can actually rebuild your bones by using light weights to build muscle and bone mass. By just moving and walking, you can take off inches without losing weight because exercise reduces fat while building muscle and bone. But muscle is heavier than fat and takes up half the space. So you might not lose weight right away, but you'll look and feel better!

There used to be a theory that each of us, after a certain age, could not increase muscle strength or muscle mass. But a group of 90-year-olds, with the help of researchers from Tufts and Harvard Universities, debunked that myth in a study in which patients at

"The Results Were Astounding!"

The Administration on Aging's *Fitness Facts for Older Americans* reports:

"At the VA Medical Center in Salt Lake City, fit men in their mid-50s were compared to inactive men in their mid-20s. Active older men had lower resting heart rates – 64 beats/minute versus 85 beats/minute for the younger men...slower heart beats in the first minute after exercise...What is more, the older men weighed an average of 166 pounds compared to 192 pounds for the younger, sedentary men.

Boston's Hebrew Rehabilitation Center lifted weights with their legs. At first the regimen was modest, but it was increased in time to test leg strength. At the end of six weeks, these 90-year-olds (with a variety of ailments and conditions) had increased their muscle strength by 180 percent! The researchers then asked the residents to return to sedentary lifestyles and found that, in one month, they had lost a third of their previous muscle strength. Moral: "If you do not use it, you *will* lose it—at any age."

Weight training, or "resistance" exercise, is as vital as aerobics because it strengthens your muscles and bones, while aerobics strengthens the lungs and heart. Remember, however, that if you work with weights, consult someone who is trained who can instruct you in their appropriate use so that, in your self-interest, you do not overdo it and end up with an injury or a hernia.

Get going on an exercise program, but be wise about it, especially if you are now a "couch potato." Check with a physician, health professional, or certified trainer *before* you start. If you do weight training, do so three times a week for 20 minutes under a trained instructor. Bending and stretching should be done every day for about 10 minutes, and aerobic exercise should last from 30 to 60 minutes three times a week (these are all guides to help you get started; you can increase these in time as you progress). When you do start, do it "by the book." In fact, three of the best books to guide you are:

- *Stretching (for everyday fitness and for running, tennis, racquetball, cycling, swimming, golf and other sports)*, by Bob Anderson (illustrated by Jean Anderson), Shelter Publications, Inc.,

Bolinas, CA (first published in 1980, now in its 35th printing, with over 2 million copies sold).

- *Fitness After 50: It's Never Too Late to Start*, by Walter H. Ettinger, Jr., M.D.; Brenda S. Mitchell, Ph.D.; and Steven N. Blair, PED, Beverly Cracom Publications, a joint venture between the Beverly Foundation and Cracom Publishing, Inc., Pasadena, CA, 1996.

- *Exercise: A Guide from the National Institute on Aging and the National Aeronautics and Space Administration*, published by the National Institute on Aging's Information Center, P.O. Box 8057, Gaithersburg, MD 20898-8057 (1-800-222-2225), an Introduction to which is available at:

  http://weboflife.arc.nasa.gov/
  exerciseandaging/home.html

The California Active Aging Project is one of the pioneers in developing outreach efforts to whole communities to promote fitness and exercise among the state's growing senior population. The California Department of Health Services (DHS), joined by the University of California at San Francisco (UCSF) Institute for Health and Aging, has formed The Physical Activity and Health Initiative (PAHI) to champion three types of outreach:

- The Community Mini-Grant Program, in which 16 communities have received $15,000 each to organize and implement "supervised physical activity self-change programs" for older adults preferring a group setting. Participants, who are personally assessed, agree to regular telephone follow-ups with a trained volunteer.

- Direct Mail Interventions in which, via comparatively low-cost direct mail which can reach large numbers of people, participants are enlisted, evaluated individually, provided support group contact, and assessed and informed periodically through pre-planned mailings.
- A series of outreach projects such as "No More Falls!," Global Embrace for Active Aging as part of the UN's International Year of Older Persons (1999), Senior Walking Survey, A Strength Training Task Force, and "Vitality in Motion," a handout developed jointly with Blue Shield of California.

For further information:
Steve Hooker, Ph.D., Director
California Active Aging Project
Physical Activity and Health Initiative
P.O. Box 942732, MS 675
Sacramento, CA 94234-7320
916-324-7758
web site: shooker@dhs.ca.gov

Resources on Exercise and Fitness

Your most important and immediate resource, as well as contact for support, is your local community: senior and civic centers, parks and recreation departments, YMCAs and YWCAs, places of worship, local universities or hospitals, and local gyms. Even local shopping malls sometimes advertise exercise, wellness, or walking programs. If you have heart disease or are prone to falling, check with your physician; there are some community centers with excellent fitness programs tailored to assist in special ways. Also, local libraries have books and tapes on exercise and aging.

For More Information:

The National Heart, Lung, and Blood Institute Information Center
P.O. Box 30105
Bethesda, MD 20824-0105
301-251-1222

American Alliance for Health, Physical Education, Recreation, and Dance (AAHPERD)
1900 Association Drive
Reston, VA 20191
800-213-7193 or 703-476-3490
web site: www.aahperd.org

AARP Health Promotion Services
601 E Street, NW
Washington, D.C. 20049
202-434-2277

Continued

American Heart Association
Public Information Department
7272 Greenville Avenue
Dallas, TX 75231-4596
214-373-6300

American College of Sports Medicine
P.O. Box 1440
Indianapolis, IN 46206-1440
317-637-9200 ext. 117

The National Institute on Aging (NIA)
NIA Information Center
P.O. Box 8057
Gaithersburg, MD 20898-8057
800-222-2225
800-222-4225 (TTY)
web site: www.aoa.dhhs.gov/aoa/pages/agepages/
exercise.html

Managing Your Meds

A recent study found that 19 percent of hospital admissions nationwide are directly related to adverse prescription drug interactions! Another study pegs the figure at 25 percent! That means from one-fifth to one-fourth of all the people in our hospitals are there because the prescription drugs they are taking react to each other, causing serious illness. How can this be?

About a third of this mismanagement is the result of forgetfulness or inattention on the part of consumers themselves. Sometimes they don't fully inform their own doctors about their medications; or they mix up their dosages or fail to follow instructions. Seniors and the elderly suffer these ill effects more than others by the mere fact that they get sick more often and require prescriptions in greater numbers.

Two-thirds of medication mismanagement could be prevented by sophisticated computer systems. But there are no regional or nationwide computer systems (yet) to warn doctors and pharmacists when patients are about to take drugs that will interact adversely. To establish such a system, people will have to consent to have their medical records stored in a computer, just as many of us do now at our own pharmacy. Up-to-date computer programs to warn of adverse reactions have existed for years, but there has been no agreement to invest the substantial sums it will take to create a large interconnected system.

Save Yourself, and Save Taxpayers, Too!

By managing your own prescriptions, you can avoid adverse drug interactions. You can prevent needless illness and pain–and save billions of dollars!

If even half of the projected savings were realized in hospital reimbursements alone, there would be enough saved to provide basic health care for every man, woman, and child in the United States!

Nine Vital Steps You Can Take

1. Use the same pharmacy for **all** your prescriptions.
2. Make a list of **all** your meds, using the names and dates of expiration on the bottles. Keep a copy of the list in your wallet or purse; give a copy to your doctor(s). Keep your list updated!
3. Ask your doctor or pharmacist to review **all** your meds, including over-the-counter drugs, vitamins, and supplements to avoid conflicts in prescriptions. And make sure your meds are current.
4. Ask your pharmacist to check that the pills in each bottle are actually the meds that are on the label (the label reflects the prescribing doctor's original medicine and dosage).
5. Organize **all** your meds by day and time to be taken (you can buy already-labeled plastic trays for this purpose).
6. Write down all adverse reactions to medications, no matter how minor. Include the time of day, what you've eaten, and which meds you have taken. Most drug interactions have only been tested for a combination of two drugs. Where three or more drugs are interacting at the same time, doctors want patients to report so that they are aware of adverse interactions.
7. Know the contraindications (side effects and restrictions) for each medicine you are taking–even vitamins!

8. Know, by asking your doctor or pharmacist, what each prescribed drug is for, what the expected results are, and when you should call to report even minor adverse reactions.

9. If there are no adverse reactions, take **all** of any individual medicine you are prescribed–unless told otherwise by your doctor–**even if you feel better**. Usually, the amount prescribed is designed to ensure that you **stay** well, particularly drugs taken for chronic conditions (such as heart disease, blood pressure, thyroid, or diabetes) over a long period. Others, such as antibiotics, need to be taken for a full course of treatment (usually 10-14 days) to prevent a recurrence of illness.

For More Information...

Contact the organization in the State of California which is the pacesetter in this field:

The SMART Coalition of California (Senior Medication Awareness and Training)
P.O. Box 188528
Sacramento, CA 95818
916-444-5401
Ms. Ellie Enriguez Peck, Program Director

A recent study by Professor J. Lyle Bootman, Ph.D., Dean of the College of Pharmacy at the University of Arizona Health Sciences Center, labeled medication mismanagement a **"$76 billion national disgrace."** (This figure includes hours of work missed due to **avoidable** hospitalizations.) Another study, this one by the National Council on Patient Information and Education, indicates that the percentage of hospital admissions from drug reactions may be higher (25 percent) than the figure used in the Bootman Study (19 percent). If that is the case, then the cost to the nation may be higher as well.

Using the latest figures available, the average cost of a day in a hospital in the United States is $1,779 (*Current Trends in Health Care Costs and Utilization*, Mutual of Omaha Companies, 1994). Multiplying this daily cost by the number of in-patient days per year (259,114,949 days—*Hospital Statistics: Emerging Trends in Hospitals*, American Hospital Association, 1996-1997 edition) brings the total annual cost of all hospitalizations in the nation to $461 billion! Based on the Bootman Study estimate, **up to $69 billion can be saved** through effective medication management. Based on the National Council on Patient Information and Education's estimate, **over $115 billion can be saved!**

Thus, effective national medication management can save not only needless hospitalizations, illnesses—and, yes, even deaths—it can also save *more than enough* money to provide every citizen with full access to health coverage.

For More Information...

The California Medical Association
P.O. Box 7690
San Francisco, CA 94120
415-541-0900

The California Pharmacists Association
1121 I Street, Suite #300
Sacramento, CA 95814
916-444-7811

Ironically, for years, women were not included in test groups for new drugs because of their cyclic hormones and childbearing capabilities. Yet, those very reasons explain why women are different from men when it comes to medication management. Only now are these differences being taken into account in testing processes. Otherwise, women become "test cases" every time a drug or combination of drugs is prescribed for them. Women, who make up the majority of seniors, must be doubly aware and report to their doctors regularly. Men produce hormones at a fairly static rate throughout their life span. Women, on the other hand, are cyclic; that is, women experience a fluctuation within the context of the hormone "cocktail."

Clearly, an acute awareness of the context in which women take medications is vital! When visiting a physician, it is essential that women know and report their time of cycle, eating and sleeping patterns, and any supplementary hormones they are taking (these supplements can increase, delay, or sometimes compete with medicines and nutrients). Why is this essential?

For example, 53 percent of women over 50 die from heart attacks, but recent reports show that estrogen use in post-menopausal women may decrease heart attack risk by half. Thus, there is an understandable urge by the medical community to "medicalize" menopause. That's why women, especially, must keep doctors informed of the full range of their medications. And that starts with **self-awareness**!

Reactions to medication are very individual and may vary within the individual from day to day. Each woman must be aware of her own body response, know what else she is ingesting, and keep her doctor informed, especially if she stops taking her medications for any reason (some must be tapered off gradually).

Men have a high proclivity for heart disease and high blood pressure. Statistics show that men have a greater risk of developing heart problems and increased blood pressure than women. While this is not alarming, it demonstrates that there are certain health conditions that men should pay attention to especially. In addition, both men and women should pay attention to this:

The incidence of prostate cancer in men is one-third greater than that of breast cancer in women!

This is NOT to say that one cancer is more alarming than another; instead, it means that the attention paid to one should be paid to both. As in the battle to prevent breast cancer, self-examination and early detection among men concerning prostate cancer are vital. Men must learn to do their own self-examination, make regular checkups with their physician a routine (if they are over 50 years of age), and use common sense. How many times have women been so admonished about breast cancer? Well, the same applies to men! (See section on "Prostate Problems and Prostate Cancer," page 270, for more information.)

Patients' Bill of Rights

Advocating for a Patients' Bill of Rights seems new because of recent debates in Congress. But, while enacting national legislation is overdue, the concept has been discussed in various venues since the American Hospital Association adopted the first Patients' Bill of Rights in 1973 (revised in October, 1992).

Some states have adopted legislation that partially codifies elements of a Patients' Bill of Rights, some of it enforceable in a court of law. Most state proposals, however, arose from the controversy surrounding managed health care, and most state legislation suggesting a Patients' Bill of Rights is generic, applicable to all health care providers for treatment of all diseases, illnesses, conditions, and chronic pain.

In truth, the movement for stating the rights of patients in clear terms has been growing in recent years—not just in the form of legislation. A quick check of the Internet under the generic query, "Patients' Bill of Rights," yields more than a dozen pages of articles, news releases, and listings. These address rights under every imaginable disease or health condition, physical or mental. It seems that every possible health care provider organization has joined in making promises to patients, and almost every academic institution has studied appropriate wording in detail.

In brief, you, the patient, without the benefit of national law, (and in the states not yet counted in this regard), have been protected only by good will. But good will must be enforceable evenly across the nation, so that it can be understood by all who are involved in patient care.

> **An Executive Memorandum**
>
> On 2/20/98 former President Bill Clinton issued a memorandum ordering federal departments that provide, or pay for, health care services to comply with his Commission's Patients' Bill of Rights.

In fact, many of the nation's health care consumers do have some protection under an executive memorandum issued by former President Clinton in February, 1998. Responding to obvious complaints, the president issued a Patients' Bill of Rights for all those covered by Medicare, Medicaid, and other federal health programs. The president, whose authority to do this by executive memorandum is being challenged, issued his memo with the compelling argument that he had the responsibility to ensure that those whose health care is paid for, in part or in whole, by federal taxpayers' dollars are given what he called "minimum" standards of protection.

But, while the president's executive memorandum covers a large number of consumers of health care, especially the elderly, it cannot cover the vast number who are insured, who have managed care coverage, or who are not insured or covered at all. And, of course, it is not yet determined that an executive memorandum to this effect is other than useful persuasion.

Commission Goals

1. Strengthen consumer confidence!
2. Reaffirm the strong relationship between patients and health care professionals!
3. Reaffirm the critical role of consumers in safeguarding their health!

One year before he issued his executive memorandum, President Clinton created a 34-member advisory commission, co-chaired by the cabinet secretaries of Labor and Health and Human Services. The commission was to advise on: (1) strengthening consumer confidence by ensuring the health care system is fair and responsive; (2) reaffirming the importance of a strong relationship between patients and their health care professionals; and (3) reaffirming the critical role consumers play in safeguarding their own health.

The commission issued its final report in March,1998. The report contained recommendations in eight categories:

- **"Information Disclosure"** to consumers by health plans, health professionals, health care facilities, and consumer assistance programs,
- **"Choice of Providers and Plans,"** including the adequacy of a provider network, women's health services, and access to specialists, transitional care, and choice of health plans,

- **"Access to Emergency Services,"**
- **"Participation in Treatment Decisions"** by patients with responsibilities spelled out in this regard for physicians and other health professionals, health plans, providers, and facilities,
- **"Respect and Nondiscrimination"** in treatment,
- **"Confidentiality of Health Information,"** including the right of the patients to review their records,
- **"Complaints and Appeals,"** including rigorous systems of internal review, and
- **"Consumer Responsibilities,"** including twelve steps that patients can take to be responsible.

Free copies of the full report are available from the Commission's web site:
www.hcqualitycommission.gov.

To obtain a printed copy of the report, call 800-732-8200, or write to: Consumer Bill of Rights, P.O. Box 2429, Columbia, MD 21045-1429.

Quackery and Fraud
Watch Out!

Where there is money to be made (and a lot of money is spent on health care), there will be scam artists and thieves who will sell you everything from "snake oil" to unproven quick cures. These are people who will take your money without a serious thought to the consequences to your health and your financial well-being.

You are your own best guardian against quackery and fraud. Don't sign anything that is a contract without checking with a family member or trusted friend. **JUST DON'T SIGN ANYTHING!** Remember, 60 percent of all victims of health care fraud are older people; this is in part because people with infirmities are desperate for hope, for cures, or for relief that is not realistic.

This is not to say that there aren't legitimate alternative forms of health care that can relieve symptoms of conditions or diseases, but you should be wary of people who suggest that they can retard or stop the aging process (some even advertise that they can reverse it). One particular target of scam artists offering false remedies is arthritis, because there is no cure for most forms of arthritis and the symptoms can come and go. So this is a case where the elderly can be an easy target, and the scam artists can even claim "success."

Another target is so-called "cancer cures"—unproven methods of treatment that can get quite involved with diets and "medicines." Some of these may do no harm to health, but they can be costly as well as worthless. It is possible, however, for proponents to argue that providing a person with hope, even if the hope has no basis in medical fact, gives a psychological boost that can enhance quality of life. They'll take your money all the while—but if you think it's worth it, it's your choice.

Look for truth in advertising. The media often screen for truth in advertising that is submitted to them, but they can't always take the time to check out claims thoroughly, and some media executives are more diligent than others. Check out products that are sold, especially door-to-door. Remember the adage: "If it's too good to be true, it probably is."

The National Institute on Aging has information about fraud on its web site: www.aoa.dhhs.gov/aoa/pages/agepages/healthqk.html and lists the following "common ploys" used by scammers:

- Promising a quick or painless cure,
- Promoting a product made from a "special" or "secret" formula, usually available through the mail and only from one sponsor,
- Presenting testimonials or case histories from "satisfied" patients,
- Advertising a product as effective for a wide variety of ailments, or
- Claiming to have the cure for a disease (such as arthritis or cancer) that is not yet understood by medical science.

In some areas of the country, there are teams of professionals (law enforcement officials, attorneys, bankers, social workers, health professionals, and people in the field of aging) who focus on quackery and fraud, including elder abuse. They exist to protect, and advocate for, elderly victims and potential victims.

Information about Quackery and Fraud

Food & Drug Administration
HFE-88
5600 Fishers Lane
Rockville, MD 20857
888-463-6332

U.S. Postal Service, Office of Criminal Investigation
Washington, DC 20260

Council of Better Business Bureaus
4200 Wilson Blvd, 8th Floor
Arlington, VA 22209

Federal Trade Commission
6th St & Penna. Ave., NW
Room 421
Washington, DC 20580
202-326-2222

Cancer Information Service
1-800-4CANCER

YOUR QUALITY OF LIFE

Keeping Mind and Body Together

For centuries philosophers have made a connection between mind and body—a connection that is now better understood. Previously, the emphasis had been less on this connection than on the advances of allopathic (mainstream) medicine.

Yet most allopathic physicians agree that peace of mind, for example, is vital to the healing process. Thus, the interaction of mind and body might have been thought of differently in the past, but now most health professionals practice "whole" healing.

There is great virtue in meditation, deep breathing, or just "stopping to smell the roses," which helps build immunities that can ward off disease.

But how many of us *do* stop or pause in our daily lives to reflect and relax? How many of us understand that the simple act of pausing to relax is strongly connected to the prevention of illness and disease? Conversely expressed, pausing to relax is as much a part of the quality of life as diet and exercise.

Why? Because we cannot deal with the issues of the body without also involving the mind.

We are not separated into compartments. As humans, we are whole persons, not simply the sum of our parts. We cannot put our parts on a shelf (at least not

---

"Your Stomach is Doing The Best It Can!"

Recently, a man in his 60s complained that his midsection was "expanding" too much. On the one hand, he was right and needed a better diet and some exercise.

But his friend joked, "Be good to your stomach; it's doing the best it can." The friend, of course, was offering appeasement, in effect saying that his "expansion" wasn't that bad, and that he had the choice to change his habits.

But the friend was also implying the reality, which is, of course, that the stomach does *not* function on its own, and that the man could make decisions on his quality of life that would be reflected in the reduction in size of his midsection. The mind and the body go together!

---

by design) and pull off the ones that we think we will need at any given time. When we go somewhere, all of our parts go with us.

Perhaps we might challenge ourselves to examine the teachings of so-called alternative medicine and select (choose!) what might be helpful and comfortable to, and for, us. This advice stretches from the obvious (relaxation, meditation) to various natural supplements used for centuries.

But "choosing" to adapt your life to alternative influences is a giant step further than acceptance—and "choosing" a degree to which you bring these influences into your life is far more personal than following the recommendations of experts.

To reflect, to contemplate, to relax, to think thoughts beyond self, to consider your inner self,

> ### A Mode of Healing
>
> "In the end I find I can't separate brain from body. Consciousness isn't just in the head. Nor is it a question of mind over body. If one takes into account the DNA directing the dance of the peptides, [the] body is the outward manifestation of the mind."
>
> Dr. Candace Pert,
> former Chief Biologist,
> National Institutes of Mental Health,
> as quoted in *Women's Bodies, Women's Wisdom* by Christiane Northrup, M.D.

to appreciate your body—all these are practices that can make you a stronger person. Of course, you can get training in meditation techniques, but you don't need to have formal training to enhance your own mind and body connection.

Energy Systems

When we use our muscles to lift or push something, we are exerting energy. If we use our minds to solve a substantial problem, we are exerting energy. Both forms of energy are functions of the same physiological being and are accompanied by biochemical reactions in our bodies. Both involve strain that can cause perspiration, and both can cause an emotional reaction (fear, for example, of not being able to accomplish the task, whether physical or mental).

One noted author on this subject is Christiane Northrup, M.D., who wrote *Women's Bodies, Women's Wisdom* (Bantam Books, 1998). While her book is focused on women's health issues, the chapter on the mind/body relationship is applicable to everyone. Dr. Northrup speaks of the "language of energy systems," suggesting that studies have long since pointed out that people who are careless, have an angry demeanor, or are depressed are more prone to accidents or may "punish" themselves. Clearly, she argues, the state of the mind can affect the body. Conversely, when we start to understand that this interaction can impact us negatively, we can see possibilities for the reverse to be true. If we can appreciate that our energies are who we are, then we can "get in touch" with how our attitudes can impact our health.

In your own self-assessment, you might have charted how you see yourself as part of a class or social group: What have you achieved in education? What are your life skills? What is your relationship with your family and your community? These are more than habits or surroundings. They are a part of your belief system. They are the beliefs that give you hope and self-esteem.

They are factors that you must have in order to consciously affect any disease or condition that can threaten your life.

Mind/Body Connections

Psychoneuroimmunology (PNI) is the study of the mind/body connection. Broken into its parts, this fifty-dollar word refers to: "psycho," or imprints on the brain; "neuro," or the body's nerve center and communications system; and "immunology," or the body's ability to fight disease. PNI tries to unlock the secrets of how mentally painful experiences in a person's life leave scars that can prompt physical reactions.

Dr. Candace Pert, former Chief Biochemist at the National Institutes of Mental Health, along with other research experts, has documented a relationship between the chemicals of the brain and receptor sites throughout the body's nerve, immune, and endocrine system cells as well as certain body parts such as the kidneys. When thoughts and emotions are strong enough, the chemicals reach the receptor sites affecting our physical bodies *directly*. This interaction can go both ways. Some of our organs and our immune system can manufacture the same chemicals, meaning that the entire body can "think" and "feel."

The common denominator of the chemicals of the brain and the chemicals of the body prompt Dr. Northrup to ask:

> "...where in the body is the mind? The answer
> is, twhe mind is located throughout the body...
> The mind can no longer be thought of as being
> confined to the brain or the intellect; it exists in
> every cell of our bodies. Every thought we

> *think... every emotion we feel has a biochemical equivalent."*

Perhaps we shouldn't dismiss the phrase, "go with your gut feeling." That phrase connotes intuition, and there has always been debate about the intellect versus intuition, invariably suggesting that the intellect is the stronger partner. Yet, stronger or weaker, intuition is as integral a part of our experience as the intellect. And intuition comes from experience, including imprints on our bodies.

For example, a rape victim suffers a physical trauma that makes a psychological imprint for the rest of his or her life. Should that person ever be threatened in a similar way again, the brain and body will work in consort to avoid that trauma. Subsequently, the same person may attain mastery of self-defense skills and counterbalance the imprint on the mind and body.

If PNI can show a connection that explains pain and suffering, it can also show that experiences and imprints that reflect healing are beneficial in like manner. If you become sick as a child and your sickness is cured, thus alleviating your suffering, then the imprint on your mind can mean that you have confidence in that process by which you were cured and your own ability to heal. This means that you think you can not only be cured again of illness, should it occur, you can be healed as well—a process well beyond that which cures.

Thoughts, Memories, and Beliefs

"Feelings and emotions are our responses to the world as we let it touch us."

John Welwood
Toward a Psychology of Awakening

There is an energetic aliveness in each of us. Whenever you interact with the world around you, you store a sensory imprint in your body and in your mind. When you "record" the sensory process mindfully, it becomes a thought. When you revisit thoughts to recreate an experience, your memory stimulates both a mental and bodily response.

Making sense, creating meaning in your life, is a very human ability. So, when you puzzle through all the stored experiences, activating the memory "tapes," you then create a meaningful belief that reflects your own understanding of the experiences. This sounds very simple, but it can lead to complications if new experiences and understandings challenge long-held or cherished beliefs.

There is the suggestion of a progression in strength from "thoughts" to "memories" to "beliefs," at least in terms of the mind/body connection.

First, there are thoughts. In the hope of something good happening, one person may say to another, "Hold a good thought for me." The party doing the asking is not asking a major commitment, just a good wish. A "thought process" suggests more focus or concentration. One person asks another for help in solving a problem—anything from a problem in mathematics to the emotional issues of a relationship. This requires varying degrees of a thought process in which information is shared, and perhaps challenged by, the asker.

Then there are memories, born of experiences that come from thoughts or thought processes. These lead to decisions from which there are results or consequences. The results or consequences frame the memories—learning experiences, both pleasant and difficult, that can have an impact on future conduct.

In terms of the mind/body connection, both thoughts and memories can lead to attitudes that affect behavior. For example, learning the ritual of a community can be an empowering experience for many people—one that gives them a sense of belonging in their daily lives not known before. But that same experience can have consequences if the "belonging" carries with it conditions that are hard to accept.

Beliefs are usually grounded in upbringing and family, community and friends, a sense of pride in accomplishments, and encouragement from others. It is "beliefs" that most impact the mind/body connection, because they are not only intellect, they are intuitive as well. For instance, studies have shown that people who have faith that God, Soul, a Higher Power, The Great Mystery, or the Universe (terms for spiritual energy) animates their lives will possess an inner guidance that can help cure and can be healing. The opposite is also true. People who have little to believe in often do not know where to turn when they are under stress. This can lead to mental depression, self-destructive behaviors and a suppression of the immune system.

The suppression of the immune system is known clinically as an "auto-immune disease." This is literally where one's own immune system, designed to protect against disease, breaks down and can attack the very body it is supposed to defend. Auto-immune diseases include rheumatoid arthritis, multiple sclerosis, thyroid diseases, lupus erythematosus, and the Epstein-Barr virus, which has been linked to chronic fatigue syndrome, gastric ulcers, and yeast-related diseases. Of those affected by auto-immune diseases, 80 percent are women.

What does this tell us about where the stress is in our society? And how does this happen? Studies show that it is not stress itself that is the direct cause of suppression of the immune system; it is the *perception* of stress. When people feel that their stress is inescapable, a hormone or chemical substance called "enkephalins" is released into the body. Enkephalins can literally numb immune system cells.

> ## *"Recontextualizing"*
>
> "The regular and 'irreversible' cycles of aging that we witness in the later stages of human life may be a product of certain assumptions about how one is supposed to grow old.
>
> "If we don't feel compelled to carry out these limiting mindsets, we might have a greater chance of replacing years of decline with years of growth and purpose."
>
> Dr. Ellen Langer, as quoted in *Women's Bodies, Women's Wisdom* by Christiane Northrup, M.D.

But memories and beliefs can also be deep reservoirs of disease prevention and good health. You don't have to be resigned to aging as negative. Don't give in to the notion that aging is nothing but aches and pains.

Of course, there are some aches and pains, but most are not permanent if you don't want them to be. If you fall for the "aches of age," you will be trapped. If you understand your memories and beliefs, you can "recontextualize" your quality of life and be far more empowered and independent.

You cannot reverse the aging process, but you can reverse some of the *effects* of aging. And if that is so, given the mind/body connection, how might you be able to affect your own health? Aren't those possibilities limitless?

Support Systems

In suggesting mind/body connections that are deep and abiding there must also be a companion suggestion that these connections are long term, not just an asset to be called on as needed. Short-term results can be vital, but what is sustainable?

If the connection between mind and body is to be a functional reality for most people, then that reality requires flexible coping skills and accessible support systems. But sustaining these changes in your life may not be easy; you may need support. While it is possible for some people to undergo transformation individually, most of us cannot do so without assistance.

You can choose from a host of support groups that are established in many communities. Many of these groups offer services at little or no cost and are available based on eligibility criteria:

Mental health clinics are available in most communities and are often available on eligibility criteria that are not income-related alone. They are supported by federal, state, and local dollars, but they often have volunteer auxiliaries that raise money for amenities and extra services that are not included in their basic programs. The growth of mental health clinics—though often not sufficient to meet demand—results from diminished emphasis on large institutional care and a desire on the part of families to have mental health support closer to home.

The Family Caregiver Alliance, founded in 1977, is now a nationwide organization, fully capable of assisting you and your family with every kind of resource reference in the growing number of communities where they have local offices. Private and nonprofit, they are mostly staffed by trained volunteers, who are your peers and who are sensitive to the needs of families. Their services include quick, reliable information and referral.

Caregiver Resource Centers, in California, which were started by the Family Caregiver Alliance, are designed to assist both you and a caregiver. The centers are a growing component of support to help give you companionship as well as physical assistance. In California the caregiver resource centers are funded by the California Department of Mental Health.

The Visiting Nurses Association is the nation's oldest health service for the home-bound (except, perhaps, when doctors made house calls). This nonprofit, volunteer-driven association, now more than 60 years old, has chapters throughout the United States. Among its in-home services, the association:

- Offers patient rehabilitation following a heart attack or stroke,
- Monitors blood sugar and blood pressure,
- Cares for ventilator-dependent patients,
- Administers antibiotics, cancer-fighting drugs and other medications,

- Changes dressings and catheters,
- Gives instructions on medications and diet,
- Assists with personal care, bathing, and walking, and
- Provides light housekeeping and meal preparation.

The association's extensive chapters bring trained nurses into the homes of the elderly who may need them on a regular basis. Their services are Medicare-certified, and their bills are paid by Medicare, Medicaid, and the nation's private insurers for those who are eligible. The cost of "non-covered visits" is paid for on a sliding fee scale, based on a family's income, and can be adjusted to meet individual family situations.

Home health care is the fastest-growing service in health care in the United States today. It is supported by the federal government and is available in every community. Usually, home health care is provided by private companies that are reimbursed by Medicare and Medicaid. It is available if you are low-income. While home health aides are trained primarily in health assistance, the contact you have with them may well be a link to your own independence and your community.

In-Home Supportive Services is a government social service available mostly to low-income frail elderly and disabled adults. The training received by IHSS workers is basic. They provide help with daily functions and upkeep. Their assistance can mean the difference between institutional dependence and community-based independence. Often, the help and attitude of IHSS workers themselves can be the mental link to a larger community. These same services are also available privately for those who may not qualify for the government program.

Independent Living Resource Centers provide information and referral on techniques, methods, and tools to live at home and function as independently as possible. Geared primarily for the younger "disabled" community (as that term is used in the Americans With Disabilities Act), these centers increasingly serve older adults who may become "disabled" as they age.

See also "Support Programs and Services" (Page 123).

For More Information...

The **Department of Mental Health** in your county or local jurisdiction

The **Visiting Nurses Association** in your county or local area

The **Department of Social Services** in your county or local area

The **Area Agency on Aging** in your local area

The Family Caregiver Alliance
690 Market Street, #600
San Francisco, CA 94104
415-434-3388
E-Mail: info@caregiver.org

Continued

Center for Healthcare Information
400 Birch Street, #112
Newport Beach, CA 92660
949-752-2335

Healing versus Curing

For the fullness of your life to be realized, you must be at peace with your past and look forward to fulfilling dreams of things yet to be accomplished in your life. This "calm" about your world will provide the kind of "healing" of which philosophers write. Healing, therefore, comes from within and goes far deeper than curing an illness or repairing wounds or breaks.

Curing is a part of healing, but healing is a power within, often unconscious, depending on beliefs and experiences. No matter what happens in a person's life, however, there is always the power (wisdom?) to choose what adverse experiences *mean*; thus, changing the patterns of life for the better.

"Be open to the messages and mysteries of your body and its symptoms. Be eager to listen and slow to judge. What you learn may have the capacity to save your life."

Christiane Northrup, M.D., Author, *Women's Bodies, Women's Wisdom*

Too often, we find ourselves admonished to control our emotions. When we are children, we release our feelings, but we do so in an adult society that disdains tears and noise. Yet, there is a world of difference between the healing abilities of those who have the confidence that, as children, they were loved and nurtured, and those whose parents were absent or uncaring. When the latter is the case, there must be a process in place that unloads the "baggage" of the past and replaces it with dreams that will enhance self-esteem. With self-esteem comes healing, which can include curing, when necessary.

But how is healing done, assuming you have the capacity to heal? First, of course, you must "listen" to your body. If mind and body are connected, then your body communicates with your mind when it needs attention. Perhaps the most outward example of this is pain.

Be receptive to the "language" of your body, and don't be judgmental. Listen, interpret, understand, and give it meaning. Trust what you are hearing or seeing; it is believable. It may be uninvited, but it is completely natural.

Says Dr. Chistiane Northrup, "For healing to occur, we must come to see that we are not so much responsible *for* our illnesses as responsible *to* them."

Re-framing Your Life

Changing the patterns of your life is a move based on discovery—primarily the discovery that your own life is full of potential that you might not have known was there. The discovery you make may arise from the healing of depression in your life, or it may come from a longing within as an opportunity to make the most of who you are and can be. Are we ever too old to re-frame our lives?

John Welwood writes, in *Toward A Psychology of Awakening*," Depression is perhaps the most widespread psychological problem in modern times, afflicting people in both chronic low-grade forms and more acute attacks that are completely debilitating...[but] the focus on simply getting rid of depression prevents us from recognizing it as a potential teacher...If we want to *heal* depression, instead of just suppressing it, we need to approach it not just as an affliction but as an opportunity to free ourselves from certain obstacles that prevent us from living more fully."[1] These are wise words applicable to everyone, the elderly especially, for it is the elderly who, often feeling old, left out, and cast aside, disproportionately suffer depression.

It may seem impossible to garner strength from depression, variously described as feelings of impermanence or loss of control, "egolessness," or pain that leads to a sense of emptiness, which can even frighten people. Welwood writes, "If we were to look more deeply into any of these experiences, it could help us awaken to the essential openness of our nature, which is the only real source of happiness and joy."

But how do you do this? In his chapter entitled "Making Friends with Emotion," Welwood warns against "...trying to stand up against a powerful wave that is heading into shore. If we resist the wave, it is indeed overwhelming." He suggests that we learn to ride the waves, instead. Life is not a series of dualistic judgments. While there are boundaries around the conduct of life, there are no fixed outlines of good and evil,

[1] From *Toward A Psychology of Awakening* by John Welwood. © 2000 by John Welwood. Reprinted by arrangement with Shambhala Publications, Inc., Boston, www.shambhala.com

no matter how much western cultures try to make clear distinctions. People have what biologist Rene Dubos calls, "basic goodness...that lies in our inner core." But that is only the tip of the iceberg. Underneath are the senses, wider and deeper. And then there are feelings and emotions. For example, reacting against the emotion of fear or anger or sadness can be worse than the primary feelings themselves. You may recall the clear voice of President Franklin Delano Roosevelt when he rallied the Congress to a Declaration of War: "We have nothing to fear but fear itself..."

Fear, anxiety, and depression often arrive when you shift identity. The familiar structure is gone, and a new one is not yet in place. When you feel the loss of something vital, or life ceases to be meaningful, there are still choices you can make to regain your footing.

Some people seek therapy, which can uncover your pattern, identify dysfunctional habits, and help you to develop new structure and meaning. Others may choose meditation, in which they relax into the emptiness—not asking for reason or structure—but embracing the energy of just "being." In meditation, one does not hold on to thoughts, but instead allows thoughts to just flow through and away. If one holds the space open and waits, eventually a new identity emerges.

The following are useful ways to re-frame your identity:

- Allow yourself to mourn what you've lost.
- Go inside yourself to find what you need to learn/remember.
- Reach closure on the past.
- Open yourself to what you want to be.
- Explore your options.

- Invite yourself to dream; be creative.

In time, a new identity will emerge—one that is more crafted by you for yourself. This is not to say that your former identity wasn't useful to you in its time; but, as you gain wisdom, the opportunity for "newness" can be exciting. Celebrate your old identity, but, at the same time, get ready for your new life.

Remember, all butterflies have a cocoon stage.

Using every skill you have, from contemplation to meditation, you can unlock the sense of depression and "become one" with your emotions. Don't let your ego get in the way or try to control your structure.

Another level of life-change, important at any age, is called "shadow-work," referring not to depression but the "dark side" of our nature. We all have a dark side, which we try to push away. Our dark side is considered antisocial, not part of our self-image. And we often pretend it doesn't exist (feelings such as hatred, rage, jealousy, greed, competition, lust, shame, or behaviors deemed wrong by society such as addiction, laziness, aggression, and dependency).

In *Romancing the Shadow: Illuminating the Dark Side of the Soul* (Ballantine Books, New York, 1997), authors Connie Zweig, Ph.D. and Steve Wolf, Ph.D. describe our shadow side as almost a third person to be "coaxed" out into recognition, where we can establish an "on-going relationship to it, thereby reducing its power to unconsciously sabotage us. Seeing it—meeting the shadow—is the important first step. Learning to live with it—romancing the shadow—is a lifelong challenge. But the rewards are profound: shadow-work enables us to alter our self-sabotaging behavior so that we can achieve a more self-directed life."[2]

The manner of dealing with our shadow side is not to construct higher moral standards; there are enough—and that avoids what each of us must do: embrace our dark side in a long-term relationship in which we are in control. We can control our dark side if we recognize that it is there and respect

> ### *Shadow-Work*
>
> "To live with shadow awareness is not an easy path, a road on which debris has been cleared and the direction lies straight ahead. Rather...we follow detours, walk into debris, groping our way through dark corridors...:
> - Stop blaming others,
> - Take responsibility,
> - Move slowly,
> - Deepen awareness,
> - Hold paradox,
> - Open our hearts,
> - Sacrifice our ideals of perfection,
> - Live the mystery."
>
> From *Romancing The Shadow*, p.9

it, not be overwhelmed by it. Carl Jung, who coined the term "shadow," said that if, in fact, "...you are aware of your shadow and control it, there is a greater morality."

Aleksandr Solzhenitsyn wrote about the "reality" of our dark side, suggesting that "...the line dividing good and evil cuts through the heart of every human being. And who is willing to destroy his own heart?"

Consider the Greek gods. Unlike the Judeo-Christian image of one God, the Greeks had many gods and goddesses who cast dark shadows that were reflective

---

[2] From *Romancing the Shadow* by Connie Zweig, Ph.D. and Steve Wolf, Ph.D. Copyright © 1997 by Connie Zweig, Ph.D. and Steve Wolf, Ph.D. Used by permission of Ballantine Books, a division of Random House, Inc.

of humans. Some acted wickedly, lustfully, angrily, and vengefully; they even committed acts that could be called crimes. Those gods, which also represented the Greek images of good as well as evil, taught the Greeks about themselves and made them examine the mixture of good and evil and resolve those issues for themselves. "Begin an honest conversation with yourself," Zweig and Wolf advise. "...as your self-knowledge grows, so will your compassion for yourself." This, they say, results in "soul, our immanent human value," about which James Hillman intoned, "soul offers an approach to life that is sacred, an orientation toward depth."

What has this got to do with you? Everything!

Whatever your age, you can re-frame your life, if you have the wisdom to choose. There are no standards for this by which you are tested, except by yourself. There are no choices that anyone other than you can make. Much of the challenge of life is to make a positive from the reality of what is perceived as a negative.

Yet even this kind of discovery, and a decision to change your life, needs facilitation. It is one thing to try to change your life, but it is quite another to know how to do that. Modern psychologists, philosophers, and teachers, following the works of Jung, and more recently, Joseph Campbell and James Hillman, point out that you must do the "inner work" that frees you to make the "journey" of your life.

Not so long ago, terms such as *inner work* and *journey* were thought to belong to the avant-garde in our society—students, young and old, who focused on the esoteric. Perhaps that was a simpler time, when good and evil seemed more clearly defined, when loyalty through troubled times, even troubled relationships, was steadfast, and when, in post-Depression and post-war years, the struggle to survive and prosper was paramount.

But these are different times: when the Vietnam War taught us that good and evil can be confused; when people shift jobs and careers in an atmo-

> **"The Power of Myth"**
>
> "We have only to follow the thread of the hero path...
> ...where we had thought to travel outward, we will come to the center of our own experience."
>
> Joseph Campbell,
> The Power of Myth,
> with Bill Moyers, Doubleday,
> New York, 1988.

sphere of buyouts and takeovers; and when marriage is no longer "...until death do us part..." because that spans many more years than it did when the phrase was crafted.

Now, even corporate CEOs go to retreats, seeking guidance from many of those same students, now teachers, who learned that inner guidance in times of insecurity is more important than making money or achieving titles. In fact, "inner work" explores how you see yourself, how others see you, how family and friends have influenced your life, and how your career has had an impact on your outlook. There are techniques for this taught by counselors and psychologists, but the analysis of these factors really requires deep thought, even meditation, before you draw your own conclusions and are then able to express them to people you trust.

In *The Soul's Code: In Search of Character and Calling* (Random House, New York, 1996), James Hillman explains his Acorn Theory. He suggests that each life is formed by a particular image—the essence of life that calls each life to its destiny. That destiny is like a mighty oak tree destined to grow from a tiny acorn. His is a liberating vision of character, desire, influence, and freedom—and a calling: "What is it, in my heart, that I must do, be and have? And why?"

Hillman writes: "...what is lost in so many lives and what must be recovered: a sense of personal calling, that there is a reason I am alive...there is a reason my unique person is here and that there are things I must attend to...that give the daily round its reason, feelings that the world somehow wants me to be here, that I am answerable to an innate image..."

"Inner work" is an honest assessment of yourself, your character, your interests, what you believe, how you show yourself to others, and, perhaps most importantly, the goals you have for your life and the people and ideals about whom you feel strongly, even passionately. There are no "right" or "wrong" answers; there are only *your* answers. And "inner work" is for everybody, even psychologists—perhaps especially psychologists.

The great psychologist Jung offered his clear and inviting insights throughout the course of his life, which ended only about forty years ago. Jung wrote a biography with Aneila Jaffe entitled *Memories, Dreams, Reflections* (Revised edition, Pantheon Books, New York, 1973). In the chapter entitled "Confrontation With The Unconscious," Jung tells of his own "inner work," describing it as "...trying to discover my own myth..." after his split with his colleague, Sigmund Freud. Jung's own metamorphosis at that time led him to write *The Undiscovered Self*, from which much of the current teaching and discussion about "inner work" and the "journey" through life is based.

Carol S. Pearson, Ph.D., has written *The Hero Within: Six Archetypes We Live By* (HarperSanFrancisco, 1998), a pathway book that explains the concept that we all have the capacity to be heroes. Dr. Pearson's book is her third edition of earlier versions now being used as texts in teaching seminars around the world. Her book includes an appendix entitled "The Heroic Myth Self-Test," a series of questions that act as a prompt to your "inner work."[3]

Her six archetypes (updated from twelve in her previous works) are the orphan, the innocent, the wanderer, the warrior, the altruist, and the magician. An archetype is a deep psychic structure or a model of inner potentiality. These inner allies can be present in our lives all at once, in balance or "cycled through" one at a time as we go on our own journey of discovery. Each of the archetypes lives within us all, to varying degrees; we are not all

Archetype	*Task*
Orphan	Survive Difficulty
Wanderer	Find Yourself
Warrior	Prove Your Worth
Altruist	Show Generosity
Innocent	Achieve Happiness
Magician	Transform Your Life

From *The Hero Within*, p.20

---

[3] To find "The Heroic Myth Self-Test," refer to *The Hero Within: Six Archtypes We Live By* by Carol S. Pearson. Copyright © 1987 by Carol S. Pearson. All quotes reprinted by permission of HarperCollins Publishers, Inc.

one or the other.

Simply stated, the orphan is a survivor, overcoming life's difficulties, adversities, and challenges. The orphan, alone but not necessarily lonely, stems from the innocent—recalling childhood, when happiness was the result of family structure and security, to the degree that they were present in your life. You can return to innocence during the course of your "journey" in the sense of achieving happiness in your life.

The wanderer is the person who risks the unknown, looking for a path that can lead to fulfillment. The warrior is the archetype of Saint George slaying the dragon—the one who battles evil and defends the good.

The altruist is a caregiver, someone who seems selfless and believes in contributing from his or her own efforts to a greater good. And the magician is a person who can transform a community, making life better for everyone.

> "In the final analysis, we count for something only because of the essential we embody, and if we do not embody that, life is wasted."
>
> C.G. Jung

In coming to consciousness within your life, you may find that you've missed awakening and living one or more of these patterns. The missing archetype may nudge its way in. For instance, someone who has always been "nice and polite" may find the opportunity to awaken the warrior or magician within.

Without the "inner work" of examining your life and direction, you may be consigned, according to Dr.

Pearson, "...to play prescribed social roles...to feel numb and experience a sense of alienation, a void, an emptiness inside." Doing this kind of self-examination may be uncomfortable for some, because it may involve the risk of discovering regrets or missed opportunities. In some cases the discovery may be the perception of negative influences that seem overwhelming. Yet, without question, at any age the risk is worth it, because the reward is a keen sense of adventure (going on your own journey), a quest for self-esteem, which results in being much more a part of your community. To deny this to yourself may mean that you are suppressing yourself in order to please others. In that case, you become what Dr. Pearson calls a "performance machine" or a "chameleon...to serve an image [that] buys success..." or just keeps you safe.

Archetype	Plot Structure	Gift
Orphan	How I suffered or how I survived	Resilience
Wanderer	How I escaped or found my own way	Independence
Warrior	How I achieved my goals or defeated my enemies	Courage
Altruist	How I gave to others or how I sacrificed	Compassion
Innocent	How I found happiness or the promised land	Faith
Magician	How I changed my world	Power

From *The Hero Within*, p. 18

Going inside yourself thoughtfully, conscientiously, and honestly will produce results that are completely authentic. In fact, your authenticity will be noticeable because you become more genuine in the eyes of others as well as yourself—not just a person who thinks he or she is *entitled* to gifts or services, even though you may graciously receive them.

Having completed enough "inner work" to decide where you want to go with who you are, you are now ready for your journey, regardless of your age, because there is always more to life—even death.

Recently, a man who had lived the life of a Tom Sawyer in his youth—a war hero, an amateur inventor, and a traveler—approached the diagnosis of a brain tumor with reflection and resolve. After the initial disbelief, he resolved to organize his life and plan his death. He examined his life, celebrated the good times and winced at the bad ones, and announced that he would make his journey his way. And he did, with the thoughtfulness of someone who was comfortable with himself, completely conscious of his decisions—even at peace with how his family and others would think of him. His journey was to leave a legacy on how to die.

The larger truth, of course, is that this was the last stage of a journey that he had been taking for some time. It's just that the circumstance of the diagnosis prompted him to assess his "in-

---

Risking Change

"One always learns one's mystery at the price of one's innocence."

Robertson Davies, *Fifth Business* [4]

---

[4] From *Fifth Business* by Robertson Davies. Copyright © 1970 by Robertson Davies. Used by permission of Viking Penguin, a division of Penguin Putnam, Inc.

ner work" one more time and to decide the balance of his journey.

Did he suffer in the process or struggle with himself? No! His was not a single heroic act, nor did he seek status he didn't already have. He didn't have to be someone greater than himself. He simply followed his own path with determination. His example was completely authentic, and it became the lesson he hoped it would be. His happiness, in the end, was the taking of the journey itself.

"The emerging heroic ideal," says Dr. Pearson, "does not see life as a challenge to be overcome, but a gift to be received." And, she warns, there will be those in your life who will oppose, even ridicule, you for your effort. They are the people who, for reasons best known to themselves, want to exercise control over your life. They even may have caregiving motives, but they are, at best, patronizing—at worst, people who fear your individualism. You have the right to seek vital nourishment for mind/body/spirit and vanquish that which saps your strength or depletes it.

Going on your own journey is a very individual experience; it is not a group exercise. In fact, groups, by definition, seek to find common ground, which is fine for the group, but may discourage you from being the complete individual you can be. Once you are on your journey, you may well become an example to the group.

The journey itself is the treasure of your life, and if it is truly your own way of life, it will never end until life itself ends. And beyond? Who knows?

Belief in yourself may stave off depression and substitute optimism as logical and coherent.

There is nothing to rec-
ommend that a glass at the
half-way mark is one that
is half empty, it is also half
full, even if there is constant drinking and pour-
ing. Depression has be-
come a national "illness,"
but there is no percentage in it.

> ### An Individual
>
> "I don't develop; I am."
>
> Pablo Picasso

If you outline your own life experiences, and list
what you concluded about them (good and bad), what
you learned from them and how those experiences have
changed your life, you will have evaluated your alternatives, understood the implications, and opted for use-
fulness, not despair. This is your own dialogue with
yourself.

Libraries and bookstores are filled with advice from
authors who have written "how-to" books. Their work
has helped hundreds of thousands of ordinary people
discover that they have potential well beyond what their
lives had been up until they were introduced to reach-
able "inner work" leading to their own life journey.
These works are being used by people from all beliefs
and backgrounds, from all over the world. There are
many choices. You must find what's right for you.

Dr. William Glasser, in his book entitled, *Choice
Theory,* outlined ten statements called "axioms," which
he thought could be guideposts along anyone's journey to a new quality of life. The axioms are thought pro-
voking, requiring you to assess their validity in your
life and either your agreement with, or modification of,
them to see if and how the axioms apply to you. Can
you recognize these statements as part of your life?

Ten Axioms of Choice Theory

From *Choice Theory:*
A New Psychology of Personal Freedom [5]
by William Glasser, M.D. (HarperCollins Publishers, 1998)

1. The only person whose behavior we can control is our own.
2. All we can give or get from other people is information.
3. All long-lasting psychological problems are relationship problems.
4. The problem relationship is also part of our present lives.
5. What happened in the past that was painful has a great deal to do with what we are today, BUT revisiting this painful past can contribute little or nothing to what we need to do now.
6. We are driven by five genetic needs: survival, love and belonging, power, freedom and fun.
7. We can satisfy these needs only by satisfying a picture, or pictures, in our quality worlds. Of all we know, what we *choose* to put into our quality worlds is the most important.
8. All behavior is total behavior and is made up of four inseparable components: acting, thinking, feeling and physiology.
9. All total behavior is designated by verbs.
10. All total behavior is chosen, but we have only total control over the acting and thinking components. We can, however, control our feelings and physiology indirectly through how we choose to act and think.

These axioms have as much to do with the "how to" of our determination to change as the decision itself. We need to seek out these "stations of change" in our own communities. There is a wealth of "us" that has yet to be expressed, notwithstanding the expressions of well-meaning family and friends who say, "You can't do this. You are too old or too frail or too diseased to accomplish anything." With due respect to them and the family they represent to you, they are misguided.

You are empowered over your own life. Make no mistake about it. To the extent you want to be, you are the master of your own destiny—no matter how late in life it may seem.

The Vision of Spiritual Eldering ®

Spiritual and *eldering* are two generic words (one a construct) which, when used together, suggest a vision about growing older that is more focused on the future than the past, and more attuned to being a continuing contributor to society than a relic. It has also become a substantial movement among social thinkers and people involved in the professional world of aging.

The founder of "Spiritual Eldering"® is Zalman Schachter-Shalomi, affectionately known by his followers as "Reb Zalman." "Reb" is a term of respect, used primarily by Orthodox Jews, to refer to a senior rabbi who has distinguished himself by possessing learned wisdom often expressed in teachings and writings that are widely recognized. If a rabbi is a teacher, then a "rebbi" is a master teacher. "Reb" is a bit of American slang, and the reference to his first name is more American license, but endearing.

Reb Zalman's "profound new vision of growing older" is set forth in his benchmark book, *From Age-ing To Sage-ing*, published in 1995 by Warner Books, New York. The book is co-authored by Ronald S. Miller, a journalist long active in writing on issues involving health and older adults. And the vision of "spiritual eldering" is promoted through the establishment of the Spiritual Eldering® Institute, headquartered in Colorado.

Reb Zalman takes his readers on a journey from the days when families and tribes in many cultures acknowledged, respected, and honored their elders as people experienced enough to dispense wisdom, to today when material goods and distractions relegate aging to a negative role, one of failure.

> ### *Harvesting Life*
>
> *"If I had to die now, what would I most regret not having done? What remains incomplete in my life?"*
>
> From Age-ing To Sage-ing,
> The Introduction

The author sees far more potential in growing older—"a badge of success," he calls it: "being a sage ...whose balanced judgement provides wisdom for the welfare of society."

He calls on each of us to harvest our past...and search for new social action, thereby giving meaning to our lives ("old age is a time for self-development and spiritual growth") and providing a service to benefit others ("making contributions and a legacy").

To be positioned for this "potentiality," you have to do the "inner work" on self-assessment, appreciation, and change to give you the tools to develop—so much so that you will feel a sense of urgency and excitement about being "...a herald of the next phases of human and global development."

Reb Zalman is not shy about his vision. He sees a global impact, particularly as the population of the world ages over the next 30 years. In his vision he sees sages, Councils of Elders, providing leadership on global environmental issues inasmuch as he sees the Earth as a living planet, frail and abused. "Creation," he says, "is both spirit and matter"—a belief not unlike that of Native Americans. He suggests this is also a Biblical view in which the harmonious seasons (the Equinox and Solstice) are rhythms of our life cycles.

Preparing for sage-ing® means self-examination, "harvesting" our lives, developing a "second maturity" (a "quantum leap"), and taking charge of our lives. Reb Zalman recommends meditation, in which you review your life and approaching death and make honest judgments about who you are, as a whole person, and keep your thoughts in a journal—literally write them down for your own benefit.

One such assessment was framed in the form of a poem by Bob Burdett who joined a writers' group after he retired and found himself trying to chart his future. His poem may reflect some worry, but in the end, his resolve announces his determination about his life. His resolve was to begin anew!

"What Now?"

Retired.
Off the treadmill.
Out of the rat-race.
Affairs in order.
Paper read.
Bills paid.
Laundry washed and folded -
It'll only take a minute to put away.
Enough time for everything -
Then some.
Too much of a good thing.
Too many crossword puzzles.
Too many naps.
Errands I used to do on the way from Point 'A' to Point 'B'
       have become major events.
Is this what it's supposed to be like?
I retired on insufficient data.
Now I'm expected to live another twenty-five years.
Almost ten thousand days.
A slow death.
Travel?
Romantic involvement?
Don't think so.
Need to do something productive,
Significant,
Meaningful,
Gratifying.
Like reinvent myself.
Start all over.

FRBurdett
Burdett, a retired accountant, is part of a writers' group in
Galveston, TX. This poem was printed in *The New York Times*,
National Report, 2/9/00. Used by permission.

To be a whole person, one must evaluate what Jung called "the four levels: sensation, feeling, intellect, and intuition." You must "encounter your own mortality" and be at peace with it, without focusing on death. In the process, you must heal your relationships, extend forgiveness to others who may have hurt you, learn satisfaction in the life you have lived, and chart for yourself your unlived life (what is yet to be), based on your experience and your assessment. There is no age at which this cannot be done. And a renewed meaning can emerge from this encounter—a sense that you can reach a "potentiality" not seen before!

Dying: The Eternity Factor

Perhaps the most difficult of these tasks is dealing with your own death and the dying process. Death is not only inevitable, it is something at which we don't fail. What's important, therefore, is not that it *will* happen, but *how* it will happen. If you are willing to think about your own death, you can make it part of your life.

Jung's advice was for us to hold imaginary dialogues with people whose counsel we seek, among other things, about how we fit in among the archetypes of society and our place in the context of history. Reb Zalman calls this "the eternity factor," and, like the Native American, he suggests a "panoramic view" of time, sun, oceans, air, sky, and the mind of man. Then you may say to yourself, "How fortunate I have been to live!"

Death: The Ritual

For those who believe in an afterlife, there is a "crossing over" in death that can be thought of as an opportunity—yes, an opportunity—to go on or go forward. But you do not have to believe in an afterlife for your life and death to have meaning to yourself and your community. You don't have to give in to death and just let death take you, but you shouldn't deny it, either. If you take responsibility for your death, then you will not lose control of your life—certainly not mentally—even if some of your physical functions have been diminished.

Just as there is a ritual for almost every important occasion

On Death and Dying

A Practical Guide to Death and Dying
By John White
Theosophical Publishing House,
Wheaton, IL, 1980.

Deathing
By Anya Foos-Graber
Nicholas-Hays, Publisher
York Beach, ME, 1989.

Death: The Final Stage of Growth
By Elisabeth Kubler-Ross, Prentice-Hall,
Englewood Cliffs, NJ, 1975.

in life, so also are there rituals connected with dying and death.

There are, of course, different kinds of rituals. There are holidays that are family occasions, especially when the holidays are focused on children. There are spur-of-the-moment rituals such as a picnic. There are rituals of prayer. There are rituals of saying good-bye, and rituals of giving. Finally, there are rituals of the seasons, in which we acknowledge the cycle of life: birth, aging, death, rebirth.

Rituals can become routine. You can develop your own "personal ritual," and make it part of your daily life. This is no less true of death as an experience of life than any other event of life.

Part of the ritual, in addition to the spiritual, is the practical. If you are truly at peace with yourself about your death, you will not have difficulty expressing what the advocate organization, Aging With Dignity of Tallahassee, Florida, (www.agingwithdignity.org) calls "The Five Wishes." These wishes are recognized as binding in law in 33 states and the District of Columbia. They were developed with the assistance of the American Bar Association under a grant from the Robert Wood Johnson Foundation. In more precise language, the five wishes let your family and health care professionals know:

1. Who you want to make health care decisions for you when you can't make them (a "Durable Power of Attorney for Health Care" [DPAHC]),
2. The kind of medical treatment you want or don't want,
3. How comfortable you want to be,
4. How you want people to treat you, and
5. What you want your loved ones to know.

There is a bill of rights for people who are dying, just as there is the concept of a patients' bill of rights. It is widely circulated, with more than 3,000 references on the Internet and more than 200 organizations that reproduce the same text.

Dying Person's Bill of Rights

I have the right to...

...be treated as a human being until I die.

...maintain a sense of hopefulness, however changing its focus may be.

...be cared for by those who can maintain a sense of hopefulness, however changing this might be.

...express my feelings and emotions about my approaching death in my own way.

...participate in decisions concerning my care.

...expect continuing medical and nursing attention, even though "cure" goals must be changed to "comfort" goals.

...not die alone.

...be free from pain.

...have my questions answered honestly.

...not be deceived.

...have help from and for my family in accepting death.

...die in peace and dignity.

...retain my individuality and not be judged for decisions that may be contrary to the beliefs of others.

...discuss and enlarge my religious and/or spiritual experiences, whatever these may mean to others.

...expect that the sanctity of the human body will be respected.

...be cared for by caring, sensitive, knowledgeable people who will attempt to understand my needs and will be able to gain some satisfaction in helping me face my death.

These "wishes" and "rights," however, emphasize your expectations of others—and you have choices in this regard that you should exercise. But "spiritual eldering" goes much further, as we have seen through Reb Zalman's book. In fact, "encountering" your mortality and dealing with death and dying ahead of time are only part of the preparation you need in order to be a mentor to others.

Mentoring Your Community: Healing the Earth

And that is where Reb Zalman wants to lead you, providing you are willing. He uses the popular term *mentoring* to suggest a life in older age where you are involved in spreading your wisdom to any number of audiences, large or small, in any number of ways. Mentoring, as that term is now popular, usually means an older person interacting with a younger person. But it's not restricted to age. He sees you doing your part to bring healing to your community, indeed, to the planet Earth.

Elders are healers with "invisible" productivity. They are the ones to provide "social

---

Guidelines for Mentoring

1. Listen with great spaciousness of heart and mind to your mentee's genuine concerns before attempting to share your wisdom.
2. Don't impose—but evoke your mentee's innate knowing.
3. Don't try to impress your mentee by claiming to be perfect; be your searching, tentative, very human self instead.

security," Reb Zalman says. His play on words is intended to show that elders can provide the "security" for "society" even more than the

> 4. Respect and call forth your mentee's uniqueness.
> 5. Recognize that, like everything else under the sun, mentoring has its seasons.
>
> From *From Age-ing To Sage-ing* by Zalman Schachter-Shalomi, pages 200-202

government can provide elders with the financial underpinning of "Social Security."

In an address to the United Nations General Assembly, Native American leader Leon Shenandoah declared, "Spiritual consciousness is the highest form of politics. Every human being has a sacred duty to protect the welfare of our Mother Earth."

INDEPENDENT LIVING: AN OUTLINE TO ASSIST IN LIFE'S FULFILLMENT

Community Resources: Connections and Gathering Places

Community is a word that means "beyond self," an association with others with similar situations and interests to whom you may choose to give of yourself and to receive in like manner. Community may be spiritual, recreational, political, charitable, or a combination of these. It may involve a few people or, in the sense of an audience, a room full of people. Most of us have a sense of community, even if it extends only to our family members; some of us feel obligations to serve as contributors to causes or a body politic. Community, a connection with others, is almost always found at gathering places (although the Internet may be changing this).

Senior Centers

Today almost every town or city of any size has a senior center or a community center at which there are activities specifically planned for older adults. The main focus is on mealtime—the noon hour—when late morning or early afternoon programs can surround a "gathering" in a dining hall.

For many, this is the main meal of the day, often provided by the congregate meals program (Title III) of the Older Americans Act. Certainly, it is the one time of day when most seniors using the center are present. Announcements are usually made, or there might be a small program in conjunction with the meal. People see friends this way every day and can compare notes on activities and interests. In many communities transportation to senior centers for meals also is provided.

Senior centers are often intergenerational when time and space allow. Programs involving younger people and older adults together are becoming more commonplace. Newer senior centers are being built near school buildings so that common open areas can be used regularly rather than sit idle for long periods of the day. This can save substantial dollars in operating costs. And with the Baby Boomer generation approaching retirement and old age with increasing demands, some cities are now budgeting for repairs and new construction of senior centers.

Places of Worship

The word *synagogue* means "gathering place." In ancient Judaism, there was but one temple—in Jerusalem—but, in time, realizing that all the people could not gather in just one place, the rabbis developed the concept, then the reality, of "synagogue." In Israel today, the ruins of some of the ancient synagogues dot the shores of Lake Tiberius, where Jesus' Sermon on the Mount is said to have taken place. The synagogues were designed differently, but all had common characteristics relating to ritual.

Ritual, of course, is vital to most people. It is a habit—even a hallmark—of community. Ritual denotes passages of time or major events in the life of an individual or community, from birth to death. And most ritual takes place in places of worship.

The United States is a society of diverse religions where there is more in common about the formation of places of worship as gathering places than that which makes them different. The same can be said of rituals, because much of the celebrations and observances of one religion are similar to others. For example, observances of the seasons are often a common feature of diverse religions.

Of course, there are differences, but when it comes to "community," you have a choice as to which one you choose to emphasize in your life. If you choose that which is in common, then your "community" is larger and has greater diversity and strength. If your choice is narrow, then, by definition, your "community" can be exclusive.

Most national organizations representing major religions are focused on the communal strength of combined missions and activities. Places of worship and related organizations can have a community reach that enriches and enlightens a wide range of individuals.

For example, their leaders, acting together, can plan programs to help the least fortunate among us or young people who need mentoring. These are programs in which you can participate to become part of a greater whole and enrich yourself at the same time. Through your own place of worship, you can find out about missions that interest you.

Interest Groups and Clubs

Are you a strong advocate for a political cause? Or a candidate for public office? Or interested in an issue that your town or city needs to address? Or…? Or…?

Do you play cards? Do you build model trains? Do you write poetry? Do you…? Do you…?

For every political cause, there is an interest group. For every hobby or recreation, there is a club. These types of community can add fulfillment to your independent lifestyle as much as senior centers or spiritual activities. In fact, many interest groups and clubs gather at these "gathering places."

Most groups conduct outreach to tell you about their cause or, in some cases, alarm you. If you think you agree with them, contact them. But, like any consumer, do your homework. Find out who is behind the group and what the full range of its cause(s) may be. You may find you agree on the issue that attracted your attention, but you may disagree about related matters. Or you may like the people you meet, yet learn that the funding behind the group comes from somebody with an axe to grind or a profit to be made. Be discerning.

If you are of a mind, run for political office. There are hundreds of local offices, from hospital boards to abatement districts, that need candidates. Or volunteer to be appointed to a city commission. Are you afraid you might not be elected or appointed? Are you concerned that you don't have a political background? If everyone were like that, we wouldn't have citizen-government. And, whether seeking elective or appointive office, you must be willing to ask for people's votes or be considered for appointment. There is no harm in asking or in competing with others if you are fair and honorable.

In his book *From Age-ing To Sage-ing*, Rabbi Zalman Schacter-Shalomi suggests environmental concerns as a mix of the spiritual and the natural world that surrounds us and implies elder counsel on everything from litter removal to action on global warming. We all have a role to play, if we will but extend ourselves, thereby giving our lives meaning and purpose.

Educational Opportunities

"Lifelong learning" is now an expression in common use. All kinds of colleges and universities are now geared to accept older adults in their classrooms—even remote (Internet) classrooms. Courses do not have to be taken for credit; many can be audited, but fees are applicable.

Community colleges are perhaps best geared to serving older adults. On every campus the demographics of those crossing from one class to the next are changing. Subjects about which you might always have been curious may be available. Or you may want to learn more about an interest you have always had. Almost all of us live now in communities far more culturally diverse than in the past. That might prompt you to want to learn a new language.

Campuses are also gathering places for all sorts of clubs, interest groups, and religious institutions. You can volunteer for a host of programs or just participate in intellectual discussion at a coffeehouse. You can avail yourself of campus cultural events or sign up for field trips.

In all of these venues, you will acquire new knowledge while perhaps even adding your own wisdom to class discussion. The traditional role of the elder in most societies is to counsel and act as a role model for the young. While you may be concerned about the tendency of some people to discriminate against the old, you can shrug that off while encouraging even your critics to see you as a vital, lively person who can provide an example for them to follow.

> ### *Lifetime Education*
>
> One "student," now in her 70s, has audited at least one course each semester or quarter since she earned her masters. Had these courses been for credit, she would have the equivalent of seven doctorates.

Most often, community college campuses are within easy driving distance, or there is public transportation available. You may even know some of the teachers. Today colleges are hiring more seniors, with professional credentials, to teach courses as an assist to the regular faculty. Look for them on campus.

Volunteering and Spiritual Fulfillment

In the spring of 1998, the California Department of Aging conducted an extensive survey to find out how many volunteers there were in its programs (Older Americans Act and Older Californians Act). The survey requested information from 525 senior centers, 107 Adult Day Health Care facilities, 22 Multipurpose Senior Services programs, 33 Ombudsman programs, and 33 local Area Agencies on Aging (see "Support Programs and Services," Page 123).

The result? There were 67,620 volunteers in the state. If California represents roughly 10 percent of the U.S. population, then, by extrapolation, it can be assumed that the number of volunteers working in Older Americans Act programs nationwide is between 650,000 and 700,000!

The California survey asked about the average hours worked in each program. The total hours worked per week in all programs was 757,120. Multiplying that by California's minimum wage at the time ($5.75/hour), the total value of those hours—per week—was $4,353,440—an annual value of $226,378,880! At the state minimum wage rate in 2001 ($6.25/hour), the per week value is $4,732,000 or $246,064,000 annually. In 2002 California's rate is $6.75/hour; that's $5,110,560 per week, or $265,749,120 per year!

The monetary value of California's volunteers—calculated at minimum wage only (to be conservative) yet knowing that 39 percent of volunteers are professionals who volunteer in nonprofessional capacities—is more than the combined federal and state appropriations for Older Americans Act and Older Californians

Act programs ($159 million in 1998-99). With these volunteers, the State of California realizes a 142 percent return on its investment.

Why all this data? To make a point in mundane monetary terms that people can understand. Value! But the value is far more in the giving of one's self and the receiving of care.

There is a spiritual expression that goes with caring enough to volunteer your time and talent. And that expression is received and appreciated, even by those who seem unable to respond. A mere touch of the hand to someone bedridden, the patience given to someone with Alzheimer's disease, the myriad tasks and support given to someone still independent at home but infirm, the sharing of your world or listening to the stories of others. These are the contacts that comprise value far greater than saving taxpayer money, as important as that might be. These are the relationships with which people account for their lives in the final analysis, far more than their jobs or professions. Volunteers who give of themselves can touch a deeper meaning in life that some didn't even know was there.

There are lots of ways to volunteer to wide varieties of people and causes. But if your interest in volunteering is to assist seniors and the elderly, contact your local Area Agency on Aging. There are more than 600 of these organizations throughout the United States. They are listed in your telephone book, usually under government headings relating to social services. You'll be very glad you did.

Support Programs and Services

The Older Americans Act (OAA) was established in 1965, the same year that Congress enacted Medicare. The leadership spark for OAA was Florida Congressman Claude Pepper, whose devotion to programs for seniors and the elderly was legend. Pepper himself, irascibly independent, died in office in his 90s.

The major theme in OAA was to establish a strong meals program, both congregate and home-delivered, to set forth a basic protection against abuse in nursing homes, and to provide a framework for advocacy for seniors' programs and services. Over the years, OAA has proven itself a major success, expanding its reach to include federal financial participation in programs through a network off 667 Area Agencies on Aging, located in every community in the nation.

In addition, most states have enacted copies of OAA, providing state authority for matching federal incentives and adding programs on their own. Too, many states have acted courageously to integrate their services so that seniors and the elderly don't have to bother with bureaucratic separations and barriers to receive a continuum of care. Oregon, Wisconsin, and New Jersey are among the states that have led this effort. They have established models of how to overcome protectively crafted streams of money that pose frustrating blockades to the merging, for example, of social and health services for the same client/patient.

All the while, OAA was proving its worth in terms of enhanced independent living for hundreds of thousands of seniors. It may have taken more than 30 years,

but for the first time in history, even as the older population grew proportionately by 18 percent, nursing home
occupancy rates went down!

This astounding conclusion was the result of the 1995
National Nursing Home Survey, conducted by the National Center for Health Statistics, a division of the Centers for Disease Control and Prevention. This survey was
the fourth in a series begun in 1974. But this survey measured the trends of a decade (1985-1995). In the previous studies, nursing home occupancy rates paralleled
the increase in the older population, the age group that
comprises 90 percent of nursing home residents.

For the 1985-1995 period, the survey showed a national nursing home occupancy rate that was 87.4 percent of the previous period. In each of the four regions
of the United States, the rates showed similar declines:

Northeastern	91.5 percent
Midwestern	87.7 percent
Southern	86.4 percent
Western	83.2 percent

When the results of the 1995 Survey were announced
by former Health and Human Services (HHS) Secretary
Donna Shalala, she said:

> "Americans who need long-term care have
> more choices today. Many more are able to
> stay in their homes and receive the care they
> need."

The HHS news release said, "She (Shalala) attributed
this shift to the rapid growth in home health care as
well as advances in medical technology that permit
people to postpone institutional care and opt for **less
costly home-based alternatives**" (emphasis added).

Those "home-based alternatives" are the services offered by the Older Americans Act and various state acts that provide congregate and in-home meals, transportation, companionship, volunteer opportunities, and adult day health care—in short, all those social services that are provided to assist seniors and the elderly to remain as independent as possible for as long as possible.

More than 30 years of investment in OAA (and related acts) is paying off—not just in dollars compared to institutionalization, but in human costs. OAA contributes to the fact that greater numbers of seniors remain in independent living, have a better quality of life, and enjoy better health. If ever a legislator was validated for his vision, it is Claude Pepper of Florida. A former senator who returned as a member of the House of Representatives, he crafted his legacy like few others have the chance to do. Now, his legacy is secure.

Area Agencies on Aging

The major administrative and funding instrument that Congressman Pepper chose to carry out the programs of OAA was a local Area Agency on Aging (AAA). In so doing, he, in effect, formed a whole new local level of government with direct federal funding. He chose not to deliver funds and services through counties or cities, but instead opted to funnel funds through the states to the AAAs. In this fashion he ensured that the funds would be used for senior services. And he ensured that there would be a cadre of experts at the local level to deliver those services.

AAAs vary in size and cultural composition. Some are governed by representatives of elected local boards. Others are elected boards. Still others are nonprofit entities with appointed governing boards. Some AAAs are small and rural, but two in California (Los Angeles County and the City of Los Angeles) have a population of seniors equal to one-third of all the seniors in the state. Still another California AAA is comprised of seven counties with a governing board made up of appointees of each of the seven elected boards of the counties. Another is the founder and agent for a major complex within its major metropolitan area where the complex combines local social service, health, and park and recreation departments with aging; thus allowing an integration of services. On the following pages are descriptions of some of the OAA programs throughout the nation.

Meal and Nutrition Programs (Title III)

The meals programs are the centerpiece of the original OAA.

Meals, always monitored by nutritionists, who are as careful with taste as with diet, are served in congregate settings (senior centers) and delivered to

---

The Ombudsman Program

Crafted as an integral part of the original Older Americans Act, the Ombudsman Program has two major purposes:

- Recruit volunteers to act as companions to those in nursing homes, especially

people living independently (in-home).

Funds are allocated to the meals programs in each AAA through the states, which distribute to the AAAs based on a formula.

The OAA meals are free to everyone, regardless of income. Donations are requested but not required. In 1998, however, people across the income spectrum donated more than $167 million throughout the nation.

Volunteers in the meals programs throughout the country are cross-trained to recognize and refer health complaints at senior centers and when delivering meals at home, where they may also observe needs repairs.

those with no families, and

- Be advocates for patients and, particularly to protect elderly and frail patients from abuse.

Volunteer training is rigorous, involving a full week, after which trainees are monitored before they get regular assignments.

Most nursing home operators understand and appreciate the work of the Ombudsman volunteers, but sometimes there can be tension when violations occur.

State Ombudsmen are appointed, but are answerable only to courts of law. This independence is maintained because of patient and investigative confidentiality.

Multipurpose Senior Services Program (MSSP) and "Linkages" Programs

These programs are so-called case management; that is, the referral of a client to a professional who is familiar with all the programs and can match them to the needs of a senior, not just once but checking back many times to monitor changes. Some prefer to say "care" management instead of "case."

The funding for MSSP is shared by the federal government and the states. "Linkages," where they are established, are state-funded.

Without "case" or "care" management, there may be little accomplished and little satisfaction. Suffice to say, for OAA programs, MSSP is the link that makes independence a reality.

Adult Day Health Care (ADHC) and Alzheimer's Resource Centers (ARCs)

While these types of programs provide activities to assist mobility and mental function, both serve very different clientele.

The ADHC is a place for caregivers to bring seniors or frail elderly for daily activities so they can go to work or simply do errands. While there are no health care services at ADHCs, staff and volunteers are trained to watch for health problems and respond quickly. Many ADHCs are located near offices or shopping areas for convenience.

Alzheimer's Resource Centers are the government companion to the chapters of the Alzheimer's Association across the nation. ARCs are like ADHCs, but they have a staff that understands Alzheimer's patients and the almost incredible patience it takes to be a caregiver. Because Alzheimer's patients tend to remember further back in the more developed stage of the disease, staff members must be sensitive to cultural nuances and native tongues.

Brown Bag Program

The Brown Bag Program requires few staff members, but armies of volunteers. Like "gleaning" programs for the poor, Brown Bag delivers groceries and sundries in brown bags to shut-in seniors. Recipients may also be getting in-home meals, so the brown bag is a supplement.

Volunteers are trained to make contact, ask pertinent questions, and observe for items that may need repair.

Health Insurance Counseling and Advocacy Program (HICAP)

HICAP volunteers often are people retired from the health care or insurance fields. The title says it all. In this world of confusion on health care plans and HMOs, HICAP volunteers, supported by a staff, straighten out the wrinkles and answer questions, mostly on the telephone. And, when appropriate, the volunteers intercede on behalf of callers.

Foster Grandparents

This program receives a lot of media attention because it is intergenerational and most often takes place in the children's wards of hospitals.

There you will find volunteers acting as grandparents to sick children who might be bewildered, were it not for a loving touch and the attention of a caregiver.

Foster Grandparents and Senior Companions are run by a national contractor paid by the federal government.

Information and Referral

I&R, in most areas, includes social service referral for all callers, regardless of age, but the vast majority of calls are from seniors. I&R is composed of professional staff trained to guide callers to resources. There's a little case management skill involved, but it's all telephonic. Many states now have toll-free 800 lines for easy access. Telephone equipment "reads" the area code and prefix of the caller and automatically connects the caller to the nearest I&R.

Senior Companions and Respite Registry

Senior Companions is a federally sponsored program managed by a federal contractor. It provides volunteers and training to act as the connection between shut-ins.

and the world around them. "Companion" can mean arranging for services, doing errands, or just plain listening. In this program all volunteers are seniors, so the companionship is at a peer level, which is vital in some cultures.

The Respite Registry is a list of volunteers who are willing to relieve a caregiver when needed. Caregiving is not only time consuming, it also drains energy and emotions. Through this program, the volunteer can provide respite to the caregiver.

For More Information...

The Administration on Aging
U.S. Department of Health & Human Services
330 Independence Avenue, S.W.
Washington, DC 20201
Web Site: www.aoainfo.gov
Eldercare Locator: 1-800-677-1116 (toll free)

The National Association of Area Agencies on Aging (N4A)
927—15th Street, N.W., 6th floor
Washington, DC 20005
202-296-8130
Web Site: www.n4a.org

The National Association of State Units on Aging (NASUA)
1225 I Street, N.W., Suite #725
Washington, DC 20005
202-898-2578
E-mail: staff@nasua.org

Or your local Area Agency on Aging (in the blue pages).

YOUR SPACE

Your Environment

Housing and Surroundings

The person you are is reflected by your surroundings—not only in how you live but also where you live. The pride you have in your home or apartment (or your room, if you are in assisted living) will return to you a better quality of life.

There is a children's story that makes the point that all of us can be neat and clean, if we choose, and that cleanliness and neatness do not depend on income. It is the story of a mouse who makes use of things discarded by people to make his furniture and decorate his hole in the wall. Thus, do your own decorative choices reflect you? Are your surroundings enjoyable, useful, affordable and easy to maintain?

More fundamental is the issue of safety in the home. The simple concern about basic safety can mean that a person living independently can remain at home longer, with modest adaptations and repairs. This is especially true of older adults, who, research shows, are more likely to live in homes that are more than 20 years old. That same research shows "...that one-third to one-half of home accidents can be prevented" (Administration on Aging: AOA Fact Sheet, "Elder Action: Home Modification and Repair:" Go to www.aoa.com, then check on Fact Sheets.

Here is a list of the most common problems, and possible solutions, associated with home safety (from the AOA Fact Sheet):

Common Problems	*Possible Solutions*
Getting in/out of the shower	Install grab bars, shower seals, or transfer benches
Slipping in the tub or shower	Install non-skid strips/ decals
Turning faucets/doorknobs	Replace with lever handles
Inadequate access to home	Install ramps
Inadequate heating/ventilation	Install insulation, storm windows, and air-condi tioner
Difficulty climbing stairs	Install handrails for support

Some of those possible solutions may seem unaffordable, but there is assistance for those with low incomes. People in rural areas can apply to the Farmers Home Administration. City and suburban dwellers can apply for assistance from their local Community Development Block Grant programs.

There are programs to assist with improvements that

Publications on Home Safety

- *Home Safety Guide for Older People: Check It Out/Fix It Up*, by Jon Pynoos & Evelyn Cohen, Serif Press, Inc., 1331 H Street, NW, Washington, DC 20005. 202-737-4650. Price: $12.50

- *Safety for Older Consumers*, published by The U.S. Consumer Product Safety Comm., Washington, DC 20207. 800-638-2772. Price: Free.

- *The DoAble Renewable Home: Making Your Home Fit Your Needs* (D12470) c/o AARP Fulfillment, Consumer Affairs, 601 E Street, NW, Washington, DC 20049. 202-972-4700. Price: Free (single copies).

---

will save energy (and provide comfort) through local welfare departments and the U.S. Department of Energy. A small portion of funds in Title III of the Older Americans Act can be used for home repair. These funds are available through local Area Agencies on Aging. Some local lenders and banks will provide a Home Equity Conversion Mortgage (HECM) using the value of your current home to convert to cash. Also, the Fair

Housing Act of 1988 (Section 6[a]) protects renters by making it illegal for landlords to refuse to let tenants make reasonable repairs if the tenants are willing to pay for those repairs themselves.

The U.S. Consumer Product Safety Commission has published a checklist that reviews every area of your home and asks you to address specific questions about your personal safety. It is available by calling 800-638-2772 (ask for Document # 701) or through the CPSC web site at www.cpsc.gov/cpscpub/pubs/701.html.

The following are essential safety tips. Check all electrical and telephone cords to make sure you won't trip over them. Secure all rugs, runners, and mats. Make sure your smoke detectors work. Check electrical outlets and switches to ensure that the wiring won't spark a fire. Make sure all light bulbs provide sufficient light. Check space heaters to make sure they are plugged in to a three-prong plug to avoid the risk of fire. Check the stability of wood-burning stoves. And review your emergency exit plan so that you know your route of escape in the event of a fast-spreading fire in your home.

Common Sense Rules to Protect Yourself When Using a Contractor

1. Ensure that the contractor is reliable; beware of door-to-door salespersons.
2. Get recommendations from friends.
3. Make sure the contractor is licensed and bonded.
4. Ask for references, and check them out.

5.   Get a written agreement on the scope of work. Have a family member or friend (or a lawyer) read the agreement.
6.   Make only a small down payment; make a final payment only *after* the project is completed.

In addition to the general safety checks, in the kitchen there are loose materials that might catch fire (towels, curtains, your own clothing). In your living room/family room, if you have a fireplace, your chimney should be "swept" (cleaned out) to prevent fire. Make sure passageways and hallways are well-lighted, especially if you have impaired eyesight.

In your bathroom, your shower or bathtub should have grab bars and non-skid mats (in other words, surfaces that are not slippery). Make certain small electrical appliances, like hairdryers, are not plugged in when not in use, and that your medications are safely stored and clearly marked. Is there a light switch at the entrance to your bathroom?

In your bedroom, admonitions about rugs and runners, electrical and telephone cords, and lighting are especially important. And if you smoke, do not smoke in or around your bed. Forty-two percent of people 65 and older involved in mattress or bedding fires die as a direct result of such fires.

Work areas such as garages, basements, workshops, and storage areas should be well-lighted, particularly so you can check fuse boxes and circuit breakers as well as the electrical cords of appliances and power tools.

And make certain that flammable liquids are tightly capped; better yet, store them outside, away from buildings.

The Consumer Product Safety Commission also has a companion checklist for fire safety. The introduction states: "The United States has one of the highest fire death and injury rates in the world...every year there are more than 500,000 residential fires...4,000 people die...[and] property losses exceed $4 billion...."

These fires are caused by supplemental home heating equipment (22 percent), cooking equipment (20 percent), materials that burn—mattresses and bedding, upholstered furniture and wearing apparel—(15 percent, about half of which are caused by cigarette lighters and matches), and flammable liquids (3 percent).

But even if you have complied with every precaution about fire, you still need an early warning system (smoke detectors) and an escape plan—one that you have rehearsed. Plan ahead!

The U.S. Consumer Product Safety Commission
CPSC Hotline: 1-800-638-CPSC

Eastern Regional Center	6 World Trade Center Vesey Street, 3rd Floor New York, NY 10048
Central Regional Center	Room 2944 230 South Dearborn Street Chicago, IL 60604

Western Regional Center	Room 245
	600 Harrison Street
	San Francisco, CA 94107

In addition to making your home safe, it is important to style it so that it is convenient and pleasing to you—a place where you can welcome others, if you choose to do so. How does your home reflect you?

Certainly, there are family pictures that provide daily reference and memories. Perhaps there are scrapbooks (if not, you can make them by getting your pictures out of the box or drawer they're stored in and make a legacy of memories). In today's world you may have a computer that gives you access via e-mail to family and friends all over the world—even new friends you haven't met.

There may be paintings that reflect your taste in art or photographs of wildlife and wilderness or cities and skylines. There may be flowers, showing your preferences for color. There may be a style of furniture that you picked out years ago. And there will be the books that tell visitors much about you just by your selections. And there are your records or CDs that demonstrate your taste in music.

Your home will say a lot about you; it is a form of self-expression, particularly if you are the kind of person who likes to decorate, make little embellishments, or move furniture around to try different arrangements. In truth, these are things you have done all your life. Why stop now, just because you are older?

Also, there are improvements you can add to your home to make your life more comfortable. Brian Donnelly launched his own company, LifeSpan Furnishings (Emeryville, California) by taking a university research design project linking the design of furniture with a quality of life experienced by older people and adults with disabilities and making it into a business.

Donnelly's work was featured in an article in the May/June, 2000, issue of *Aging Today*, published by the American Society on Aging. [1] He tells how he watched his own father struggle with the simple act of sitting in a straight-back chair.

So he designed a chair with a "...high degree of leverage, stability and security in the process of sitting down or rising from a seated position. Functionally, the solution was quite simple," Donnelly wrote. "I created an arm

> **Lifespan Furnishings, LLC**
> 5901 Christie Avenue
> Suite #101
> Emeryville, CA 94608
> 800-741-9912
> Web site:
> www.lifespanfurnishings.com

that extended beyond the front edge of a chair seat and extended the chair leg forward the same distance to maximize stability. The real challenge was to incorporate these features in a way that was attractive, not awkward-looking." Today, Donnelly makes chairs and special tables. He has won seven design awards and continues his research at San Francisco State University.

Products like Donnelly's can make a difference in your life, giving you greater comfort and quality of life. Most of us will experience back pain at some point in

---

[1] Reprinted with permission from *Aging Today*, newspaper of the American Society on Aging, 21:3, May/June 2000, pp. 13. Copyright © 2000, American Society on Aging, San Francisco, California. www.asaging.org

our aging process. Furnishings that are designed for relief of that pain may well be vital to your life.

Gardening and Pets

Connie Goldman, a producer of public radio programs, has written a book called, *Tending the Earth, Mending the Spirit: The Healing Gifts of Gardening* (Hazelden, Center City, MN, 2000.) [2] Her words about gardening are spiritual:

> "We are not the same person at 40 that we were at 20. Our world looks a lot different at 60 than it does at 30. Our relationship to the garden changes, too, as we age. This simple truth has helped convince me that the enduring cycles of a garden's life—growth and change, death and rebirth—reflect the seasons of a gardener's life as well. What we observe in our gardens we also see in ourselves. I know I will grow old and die, just as surely as my geraniums.
>
> "The seasonal changes that visit my plants teach me about acceptance, patience, faith and perseverance through the travails and triumphs that are revealed in nature. In the course of a year, I see the entire cycle of life, from birth to death and back again."

Gardens, of course, can be any size—from a large plot of flowers and vegetables to a window box or bonsai—all requiring tender care, all teaching life's lessons. Considering how important vegetables are in the diet, the person who tends a vegetable garden reaps the benefits personally (and gets to grow the vegetables he/she likes).

---

[2] From *Tending the Earth, Mending the Spirit* by Connie Goldman and Richard Mahler. Copyright © 2000 by Connie Goldman and Richard Mahler. Reprinted by permission of Hazelden Foundation, Center City, MN.

Flowers not only decorate your home, but they also can be your gifts to others. More importantly, a garden can be a source of exercise for you and provide you with a sense of accomplishment and solace. "In the course of my conversations with gardeners," writes Goldman, "I've found that...what matters is how people choose to make use of this spiritual connection in their daily lives."

Goldman references her fellow author, Betty Sue Eaton (*Listening to the Garden Grow: Finding Miracles in Daily Life*, Stillpoint Publishing, Walpole, NH, 1996). "A garden is God's metaphor for life," Eaton writes. "It has its seasons, just as we do. If we look and imitate what the garden does, our seasons will pass with as fine a rhythm as the garden's."

Whereas gardens can provide solace, pets can provide love and devotion. There is the true story of a dog in England who was inseparable from his

> "The garden provided solace. It was now much more than a hobby; it became an actual connection between me and nature and God. The garden became something like a chapel."
>
> Betty Sue Eaton

master during life. After the master died, the dog would travel to the master's grave every day at dawn, rain or shine, and lay on the master's grave. At nightfall, he would return home. The dog obeyed this instinctive ritual for years, until finally, at 14, the dog died. Friends buried the dog next to his master. Then, the two were inseparable in death.

What the story reflects, of course, is the unconditional love of a pet (yes, even cats, although they're a little more stand-off-ish). We don't have to do anything to command that love, except give the animal a little attention. And most pet owners give much more than that. Our pets depend on us to be faithful; we depend on them to give us some life we would not otherwise have. It is difficult for older adults to see the cavalier treatment of an animal by some who regard pets as little more than possessions. Disregard, or, worse, abuse and cruelty are undeserved, whatever the reason. This is especially poignant, for example, for a person who is disabled or elderly and who depends on a pet for companionship or for support in performing daily activities. Can you imagine a person who is blind and who relies on a seeing-eye dog being unmoved by someone's abuse of another dog?

While the most common pets are dogs and cats, research has shown that people in institutions prefer birds such as parakeets. In such settings, birds become conversation pieces—pets to be watched and admired and whose antics can be amusing. Birds, of course, require only modest care (even if they are messy), care that can often be provided by residents themselves. In a growing number of institutions, volunteers bring in dogs that are specially selected for their mild manner and trained to be respectful.

Pets give us an energy and focus that reaps benefits in our health. There is solid research to demonstrate that pets can help prolong life and provide enhancement to a quality of life.

How You Feel About Yourself

Your environment is, of course, more than the place you live or the garden that gives you comfort or the pet that gives you energy. It is what you wear, the people you meet, the scenes you see, the sounds you hear, the weather you feel.

John Denver's song "Sunshine" was popular not only because of the music and the singer—it was the words he wrote: "Sunshine on my shoulder makes me happy…." That's such a simple statement, but it rings true. Is there anyone who hasn't felt the warmth of the sun and experienced the life-giving strength of its rays? Conversely, we think of rainy days, wishing they would go away, yet the truth is that the rain is as life-giving as the sun.

Weather *does* affect us; our moods often change with the changing weather. We check on the weather every day, and there are few topics that command conversation as much as the weather. There are retired couples who design their retirement to "follow the sun," even on a low-cost budget. And there are those who travel at times when the weather isn't too hot or too cold.

Invariably, the weather is our environment—part of the expanded view of the world that Reb Zalman Schacter-Shalomi, in his book, *From Age-ing To Sage-ing*, asks us to embrace (see "Spiritual Eldering"®). Reb Zalman wants us to include within our reach "the air, the oceans, the sky and the mind of man." He sees the planet Earth as fragile and wants us to consider an environmental postulate, much like Native Americans understood that mind and nature are one. Thus, the weather can be everything from "sunshine on your shoulder" to a spiritual awakening.

From weather to sounds to sights to the clothes you wear, the food you eat, and the places you go, you are surrounding yourself with choices—choices that enhance who you are and teach you new lessons.

Your environment is all-inclusive and can't be separated from your life. It is the air you breathe, the water you drink—it is your health. For your health to be whole, therefore, you must pay attention to your surroundings and appreciate what they give you and the choices you make so that you feel good about yourself.

Family and Friends

If you check the "Living To 100 Life Expectancy Calculator" (see page 23), you will note that one of the major criteria for centenarians is the closeness of family. Given that the researchers in that study based their formula on interviews with New Englanders who had reached 100, the importance of family was a reflection of what the centenarians considered important.

This emphasis might seem contradictory to today's world of the non-nuclear family, where communication seems to flow at the speed of light, and travel puts every corner of the globe in reach. But it isn't. In fact, the speed of communication can enhance contact and a sense of community, even around the globe and across arbitrary cultural boundaries, yielding an even greater variety of life.

It might also be true that the definition of *family* has changed. In one sense, our "families" have become more global, because the Internet puts us in direct contact with thousands of people all over the world. Today people can enter our lives through cyberspace, giving us "connectivity" that is interactive, albeit less personal than that of nearby friends. We can join groups that use the Internet to discuss everything from Jung to Judge Judy; but unless we possess the sophisticated equipment, we may not see or hear our counterparts. The use of this technology needs to be more widespread.

Vital to our future, however, is an understanding that "family" now includes friends who may be closer to us than our relatives. You recall the old saying about choosing our friends, but not being able to choose our relatives. It's true! Thus, friends can be as much "family" as family. It depends on you.

Place yourself in the context of "community"—even allowing yourself to be spiritual about it. Whom do you see as "community"? In *From Age-ing To Sage-ing*, the author asks specifically that each of us consider the Native American concept that nature and the human environment are intertwined, and that each of us can do our part to bring that harmony to light. That harmony can be pursued from a wheelchair or a mountaintop—but it is achieved through "community"—a sense of being part of a larger purpose, a sense of being, as an individual, an expression to others or a contributor to a group mission.

What are your goals for yourself? What is your mission in life?

With whom will you make your goals and your mission a "community"? Who are the family and friends who will lead you (or join you) in your quest for a long and useful life? Who are the people who inspire you to reach further in your life than you have thought possible until now? They are there! With providence, you will find them and evolve a relationship that provides meaning and purpose to your life.

Entertainment and Recreation

Take your time. You may think that, as you age, your time grows shorter (and you don't know by how much), so you will fill all your time with activities—sign up for *everything*. But even if you are energetic—and that's good—you should channel your energies to enjoy their full value. Are there any of us who have not stopped in our younger years and craved the time we have now for reflection? Well, you can heed the voice within you of your younger years. You can relax and reflect, and become a better part of your "community" because of it.

Who can doubt that we become better mentors if we pause to think through a problem, rather than suggest authoritatively that we know the answers through experience? If experience teaches us anything, it is to pause, reflect, think—then advise. The councils of elders used by Native Americans provided a forum for this, and, as a result, they were respected.

What is it that nourishes these "pauses"? There is, of course, a myriad of intellectual pursuits and just plain entertainment that can feed your interests and, at the same time, provide a sense of community. If you are an avid reader, books will provide enrichment of your interests, but they can also put you in touch with others who have similar interests.

Similarly, there are magazines for every possible pursuit in life—with magazine articles that can not only inform but also provide references (including instant web sites and e-mail addresses) so you can connect with the people and resources that interest you. In the same fashion, newspapers inform, and, with feature stories, can capture your interest in local public affairs.

What are your hobbies, and how might they fit into a sense of purpose in life? A recently widowed woman who was gifted at arts and crafts found that the time she had devoted to making Christmas presents for her family could be used to make crafts that could be sold to raise money for local charities she favored. The garage that used to belong to her late husband's tools and treasured collections of a lifetime was transformed into her studio.

Because she had arthritis, she created an atmosphere where the charities would come to her to collect what she had made, and she made tea or served wine for their visits. Visitors to her home would ask about her studio and she would show it off with pride. She always used to say that she would not live beyond a few years. She's now in her 70s and entertaining visitors each day of her extended life.

AARP

AARP (now goes by its initials only, which formerly stood for the American Association of Retired Persons) is the nation's most recognized organization for seniors.

It is an information and education, advocacy, and community services network of state and local chapters supported by tens of thousands of volunteers throughout the nation.

AARP offers its millions of members a wide range of services:
- Member Discounts (airlines, hotels, car rentals, online services, etc.)
- Member Services (insurance, mutual funds, pharmacy purchases, etc.)
- *Modern Maturity* magazine (articles on the experience and opportunities of aging)
- The AARP Bulletin (a monthly newsletter)

From www.aarp.org

A recent article in *The New York Times* marveled at the ingenuity of a group of Galveston, Texas, seniors ("National Report," February 9, 2000, Page A12) who had formed a writers' group that met at a local library to read and listen to the poetry and prose of their members.

Stories ranged from a life experience to poems that addressed the deep issues of life and death. In some sense, each of the participants wanted to leave a legacy. Although their departure from Earth was not imminent, it was important to provide a written "gift" to families, if not publishers. There, at a local library, they shared stories and opinions and reflected on their lives so that others might live. There they told of sorrows and success in the same stories.

As in any hobby or interest worth pursuing, you explore self. In *The New York Times* article, Thomas R. Cole, professor of humanities in medicine at the Institute for the Medical Humanities, University of Texas, is quoted as saying, "You can't just ask people for their happy memories. You've got to find out what's stuck in [their] craw. It takes courage."

One of Cole's graduate students, Kate de Medeiros, writes from her experience with the group, "No one, regardless of what they did for a living, ever writes about their jobs, or their weddings, or the birth of their children, or the war 'things' that many people would assume most older folks would write about...they write about [their] relationships and the very small gestures that have made them human."

Where are you in this scene? Might you not share of yourself? If your talent is writing poetry or prose, you may have an outlet in your community. What about the history of your community? Perhaps there are stories about others that should be researched and presented as part of the legacy of others.

With all the misgivings you may have about the Internet, you can glean many stories and much information from cyberspace. It doesn't take sophisticated equipment. In fact, e-mail and the Internet can be hooked to an ordinary television screen. In an instant, like millions of seniors, you can be connected with your grandchildren by e-mail—and if you are lucky to have a son or daughter who is "computer savvy," you can have instant pictures and voice playbacks of your grandchildren almost every day. And it's on your TV screen!

Shopping on-line! Now there is an experience most seniors haven't had. (Or *have* they?) According to a December 20, 1999, article by *Salon Technology* senior writer Janelle Brown, the on-line senior community is growing faster than that of teenagers. She cited data from

Jupiter Communications that pegged the number of seniors on-line at 13.7 million, compared to 11 million teens.

Excerpts from *Share Your Life Story, Baby*
By Eleanor Porter, 75

"Proms are the presumably necessary rituals of the tribe, the trials by which the tribe sorts out the most obvious winners of the most obvious stakes: the sexual stakes. The hero athlete and the pretty cheerleader. Winners in the competition of reproductive genes. Proms do not measure intelligence, sensitivty, artistic merit, moral awareness, etc....

"In the sexual stakes game, I was lost and wandering. Try, in Galveston, Texas, in the south of the U.S. of A., in circa 1939, try being female, intense, bright, anxious and too tall. Then try making small talk in spaces between partner dances. Try, hell.

"It's like not knowing how to groom, if you are a chimpanzee. You are out of it and the tall, bright chimpanzee felt therefore repeatedly humiliated and repeatedly helpless...

"...And then, a thousand years later, you are free at last. You have been loved, you have cried, you have been happy, you have lost, you have been in it and now you have personally influenced a dozen people to come to ... this tiny spot to relax and jam...

"...We are suddenly dancing free form, alone and together. We don't need partners. We are maturely sexual. We have evolved. First apes, then primitive man, then fast forward to the prom.

Continued

"And then there is Ellie, a certain female of the tribe, observed by anthropologists to have been uncertain and sad at former rituals in the early years. She is observed screaming with wine-induced laughter, free at last, moving toward death with the happy beat. Moving on. Moving on, baby. Moving."

Of the Galveston writer's group, Eleanor Porter says, "This morning, as I was getting up, some lines came to me from a play. I thought it was 'Death of a Salesman.' They go something like this. 'Attention. Attention must be paid to this man. He must not be allowed to drop into his grave like a dog.'

"And I found myself thinking: That's what we are doing. We are paying attention to ourselves. We are paying attention to our lives. To what we have done and been and lived through."

Used by permission of the author

In her article, Brown told of two start-ups, Smartshop.com and Surfree.com, a national ISP, that go around to senior centers, teaching audiences how to research products, choose on-line shops, and fill out e-commerce forms. And, while the start-ups, of course, hope they'll get their share of the business (they also give the centers computers for the new shoppers to use), they *do* make the point that seniors may find it easier to shop on-line than to go to the local shopping center.

Cyberspace notwithstanding, what about the arts and music within your locale—and who are the friends you might invite? Are you a classical music or opera buff? If so, in most communities there are ample stage shows, even travelling professional shows, to keep you on a busy social calendar—even if you are disabled.

Consider: An evening with a friend at the theater is a treasure that can lead to a late dinner and conversation. Are there other opportunities, such as museums, craft shows, county fairs, community theater, or local Broadway repeats (even at the local high school) that might give you an evening out with friends you would not otherwise have?

And what about travel—short trips with friends that can satisfy your curiosity and give you companionship? There are always the (not so inexpensive) three-day cruises to places in Mexico (out of Long Beach, California) and the Caribbean (out of Miami or Fort Lauderdale, Florida).

But travel is in the eye of the beholder. There are those who are comfortable in a sleeping bag on the ground along the Appalachian Trail or in a three-sided lean-to along the John Muir Trail in the Sierras. And there are all kinds of driving trips to satisfy every taste.

There was even one man who wanted to travel to the center of Death Valley in the heat of the summer. Aside from the fact that his family worried about him, he did what he wanted to do and boasted of his experience for a lifetime. He had no health problems at the time, so who among us would have told him he shouldn't go?

Outfit a van and travel the national parks. Get a 5th wheel and camp throughout the country, meeting fellow travelers along the way. Or live for three- or four-month periods in rentals that are the cottages you have dreamed about, if you can afford it.

If you can afford more, travel to foreign destinations and learn about the mysteries of the Nile, or the cathedrals of Europe. Travel to countries with exotic cultures and bring back wonderful memories and stories.

Make the world around you your own unique experience—whether it's a driving trip to a museum or a journey to some far-off place.

The common theme in these suggestions is crafting and living your own adventures. Planning these outings, it is said, is half the fun. There are thousands of suggestions—near and far—and at all

Elderhostel

Elderhostel can be your pathway to educational adventures (adults 55+) as close as your local college campus or on trips abroad.

Elderhostel's programs are short, affordable, and fun. And they can provide you with a new sense of community. The programs consist of classes, field trips, and social activities. (Group size is about 30).

In 1999, Elderhostel served almost 175,000 people. It has served more than 1 million people in its 25 years of existence.

U.S. program options:
- Arts and crafts
- Bicycling trips
- Intensive study
- Intergenerational activities
- Signature Cities
- Performances
- Train trips

International options:
- Classes w/experts
- Outdoor walks, treks and on shipboard
- Summer academies
- Independent studies

From www.elderhostel.org

ranges of cost (down to no cost) in books and on the Internet.

What do you have to lose? And if you take your trip with a "community" of people, what do you have to gain? Your choices are as wide, as broad, as visual, and as exciting as the world you can make for yourself.

Grandparenting...

Grandparenting linked primarily with presents and toys risks emphasizing the least, unless one of the gifts is the gift of self. The value of grandparenting relationships stems from the ongoing presence of stable, resourceful, older individuals in a younger, more erratic atmosphere where grandchildren are growing into young adults.

While a younger person tries out a variety of behaviors, identities, and explorative enthusiasms, an older person who has "seen it all" over the course of several generations can channel, reflect, and present appropriate alternatives for the child to explore. Toys and gifts that stimulate or encourage appropriate growth (books, sports equipment, the funding of lessons or trips) are all valuable connections to this role.

Providing an expensive, but necessary, item of clothing like a good winter coat, which could be a "budget-breaker" in a young family, is a wonderful gift from which parents will also benefit. And when that warm coat is linked to a few "field trips" with Grandfather or Grandmother to the great outdoors and beyond, the gift becomes priceless.

Any skill the grandparent is proud of (cooking, woodworking, swimming) can be shared and linked to the grandchild's interest. Trips to the library are free and yield great resources. Cooking can be a shared activity and a science lesson. The spending of parallel, unstructured time yields a special kind of camaraderie.

One of the greatest gifts a grandparent can provide is being a witness to the emerging personality and identity of a grandchild. Kids will try on a variety of postures, phrases, styles of clothing, and expression. Manners, posture, facial expressions, cultural awareness, and respect for others are all "free" but speak volumes about the individual. They are also learned behaviors, so our ability to model them for our grandchildren is important.

Every child has a unique sense of humor. One child will giggle at an animal that has an unexpected color (a purple cow); another loves the quirkiness of word play (poems or puns). Another child relishes physical comedy (pratfalls or "hide 'n seek"), while yet another cherishes the wink of a shared confidence. If a quiet child is overwhelmed in a huge family, moments of peace can be a treasure, but a hyperactive dynamo may need outlets in physical pursuits. With the benefit of the "long view," a grandparent's patience and creative gift-giving, which helps each child discover his or her own unique self, is the best possible legacy.

If you have no grandchildren of your own, you can "adopt" some. The Foster Grandparents Program (see "Support Programs and Services," Page 123) or volunteering in schools and youth organizations all offer opportunities for shared activities. Or you can enroll as a mentor in any one of the thousands of local mentoring programs—programs that can link you to an individual child or student with whom you meet once or twice a week.

... And Grandparents As Parents

But what if you live with your grandchildren and are raising them on your own as their legal guardian? Or what if you live in a multi-generational household with one or more of the parents?

What if you are a regular caregiver to a grandchild or grandchildren who live in a separate household? These, and individual situations like them, are a growing phenomenon in our society. A fact sheet on grandparents acting as parents was issued by Generations United.

Generations United is a national group promoting inter-generational policy, programs, and issues (202-662-4283 or website: www.gu.org—click on "resources," then "grandparents.")

According to the 1998 Bureau of the Census Current Population Survey, "...there were 2.5 million grandparent-headed families with or without par-

---

Factors In the Increase of Grandparents as Parents

- Substance Abuse
- Incarceration
- Mental Illness
- Teenage Pregnancy
- Death of a Parent
- Child Abuse or Neglect
- Abandonment
- HIV/AIDS
- Unemployment
- Divorce
- Family Violence
- Poverty

From "Generations United," a national coalition

ents present. Together, these families cared for over 3.9 million children or 5.6% of all children."

The greatest increase in grandparents as parents (1990 to 1998) was among grandparent-headed households with no parents (53 percent).

The implications these data raise for policy issues involving health care, education, and housing are huge, not to mention the legal

> ### Grandparents as Parents Are Young: So Are the Children (1996 data)
>
> - 19 percent of these grandparents are over 65,
> - 48 percent are between 50-64, and
> - 33 percent are under 50.
> - 52 percent of children living in grandparent – headed households are under the age of 6.

issues faced by the grandparents. Yet most grandparents acting as parents are living in poverty (60 percent), and most are minorities (53.9 percent, compared to 43.6 percent for white non-Hispanics).

Many communities have developed resource books for grandparents and other relatives to use in raising their grandchildren. Usually, the focus of the books is on the children, not the grandparents, so look for these books under the heading *Children*. All books include references.

The Kinship Care Resource Book, compiled by the Grandparent Caregiver Resource Center of Catholic Charities of Santa Clara County, California, hits the high points. Another example is a joint publication of The

Aging Services Division and the Division of Children and Family Services in the Department of Human Services in Oklahoma entitled *Starting Points for Grandparents Raising Grandchildren.*

These books cover government and nonprofit resources, legal issues, financial issues, medical coverage issues, psychological issues, access to child care, and issues relating to schooling, respite, and recreation programs. Enrolling procedures for child care or school can be daunting; but there is help, and there are support groups. You are not alone.

For More Information...

The AARP Grandparent Information Center
601 E Street, NW
Washington, D.C. 20049
202-434-2296

R.O.C.K.I.N.G., Inc.
(Raising Our Children's Kids:
An Intergenerational Network of Grandparenting)
P.O. Box 96
Niles, MI 49102
616-683-9038

National Coalition of Grandparents (NCOG)
137 Larkin Street
Madison, WI 53705
608-238-8751

Continued

Generations United
440 First Street, N.W., Suite #480
Washington, D.C. 20001
202-662-4283
web site: http://www.gu.org

The Brookdale Foundation Group
(community grants for resource organizations)
126 East 56th Street
New York, NY 10022
212-308-7355
E-Mail: BkdlFdn@aol.com
web site: http://www.ewol.com/Brookdale

**The Beatitudes Center for Developing Older Adult
Resources**
555 West Glendale Avenue
Phoenix, AZ 85021-8799
602-274-5022

Your Financial Security

The strong emphasis on the spiritual aspects of your life and the quality of the life that you choose are, of necessity, accompanied by the practicality of financial sustenance. That is quite fundamental.

It is axiomatic that "money helps," even if it may not be the primary force in your life. When you look for financial security, you are really striving toward that time when the necessities of life (food, shelter, clothing, etc.) are guaranteed so that you are able to opt for whatever added quality you can afford.

Consider that, when that time has arrived in your life, you are free to choose options that interest you— options that are not related to a job or basic income. You are then able to concentrate on a quality of life that allows you to try to realize your potential, but within your means. For example, you might have options for travel, from an ocean cruise to a camping trip. What suits you and your income? If you're a cruise kind of person and can afford it, go for it. If your income and interests are more along the lines of camping, go for that with the same gusto. Both are your quality of life.

Thus, your income doesn't have to be that of a millionaire in order to enjoy your own quality of life at a level you can afford. But it is vital for you to know that your income must sustain a basic quality of life so that you remain independent from institutional living and in good health for as long as possible.

Retirement or "older adult" income is a combination of Social Security, retirement systems, and savings or investments. Retirement is also affordable if your cost of living is reduced. For example, if you have paid off the mortgage on your home by the time you retire, then you won't have to pay a mortgage (or rent). That leaves you with more disposable income for other priorities.

Tax issues are always a factor for older adults in calculating retirement. For example, if, during your employment, you can defer some of your income to be paid to you after you retire, you will not only have saved that additional amount, you will have ensured that your deferred compensation is taxed at your lower rate of taxation—after you retire. The same is true of 401(k) and

IRA investments, the dividends on which can be paid after retirement.

Retirement planning is not just a casual exercise. That's why there are teams of financial planners in almost every community who can help you. Their modest fees are well worth the advice they can give you to maximize your income and minimize your outgo. Even if you think your income level is not high or that your sources of income are few, you will want professional advice, simply because experts who study financial planning are aware of techniques that you may not have considered.

Social Security

The Social Security System is a $400 billion-a-year basic retirement guarantee established in 1935. The original concept was to ensure that everyone who had been employed (qualifying by working at least 24 quarters) would receive a monthly annuity after retirement that would ensure basic sustenance. Workers and their employers would contribute to the Social Security Trust Fund out of each paycheck (6.2 percent each), and there would be enough money in the Fund to pay a monthly retirement to recipients as long as they lived. Government actuaries calculated that the work force at that

---

**Social Security Facts:
Trust Fund Income**

- Employer/employee payroll taxes (87 percent)
- Interest on reserves (11 percent)
- Taxes on benefits (2 percent)

time was sufficient to "contribute" what was paid out.

Over the years, however, the concept has been tested—not because it was a "false promise," but because Congress added some additional beneficiaries (for example, Survivors Insurance, 1939; Disability Insurance in the 1950s; and COLAs in the 1970s), which placed added strain on the fund. In addition, the demographics of the United States changed dramatically. The population aged, and birth rates declined—a combination that increased demand on the Social Security fund while diminishing the number of contributors.

> *Who Pays; Who Gets*
> - 147 million workers pay into Social Security
> - 44.6 million people receive benefits
> - 3.3 workers pay into the fund to support each beneficiary (in 1950, it was 16.5; by 2075, it will be 1.9)

Typically, members of Congress and the media, in their eagerness to sound warnings or to inform, more often succeed in needlessly scaring Social Security recipients and future beneficiaries. It is axiomatic that the same politicians who run for office by appealing to greater numbers of older workers and retirees (and who are elected, in part, because of that appeal) would find themselves out of office and disgraced if they ever let the Social Security Trust Fund become insolvent. In fact, several times in our history (most recently in 1985) elected officials have modified the Social Security Act to add balance to the books and to extend the fund's solvency for years into the future. Congress and the president will do it again.

In 2000 and beyond, Social Security has become a political issue, largely because of the media scare. Both major political parties have proposals on the table, each designed to ensure solvency while expanding individual benefits. The particular elements of these proposals, while important, are not as significant as the fact that both

> ### Payroll Taxes
>
> - "Four of five taxpayers now pay more in payroll taxes than income taxes."
> - "The Social Security tax is 'regressive.' Unlike the 'progressive' income tax, which takes the biggest percentage bite out of the wealthiest taxpayers, the payroll tax burden is the least onerous for the rich."
> - Social Security is...really a pay-as-you-go system in which current workers pay for current retirees benefits."
>
> Copyright 1999, USA TODAY
> Reprinted with permission

parties are aware of the facts and have debatable plans to move Social Security forward. That bodes well for the future of the fund. Those younger Americans who complain that the Social Security might not be there for them ought to study its history.

It should be noted that because of the American economy's long, sustained growth in the 1990s, former President Bill Clinton announced in June, 2000, that new figures put the 10-year budget surplus at $1.87 trillion. At the time, he said the nation's $3.5 trillion publicly held debt could be eliminated by 2012, and that the Social Security Trust Fund would be solvent to the year

2063, even if future Congresses and presidents did nothing to extend its life.

But politicians are always debating Social Security—if not the solvency of its fund, then the manner of investing its funds. And Congress and the president have habitually used Social Security Trust Fund surpluses to pay for other government programs, which means that the fund has not built up the capacity to sustain the kind of demand that the Baby Boomer generation may place on it in the next several decades. That's why there have been calls by some members of Congress to "lock up" the Social Security Fund, meaning that it should be dedicated only to the purpose for which it was originally intended.

In a folder entitled "Making Sense of Social Security" (prepared by Americans Discuss Social Security, a project funded by The Pew Charitable Trusts) there are nine major options for reform, any one of which could drain or add billions to the fund. The options are:

- Raise the retirement age (already scheduled to rise gradually to 67) at which a beneficiary can receive full benefits.
- Increase payroll tax rates (as of 1998, employees and employers now pay 6.2 percent each on earned income up to $68,400.)
- Invest some of the trust fund assets in private markets (they are currently invested in U.S. Treasury securities only).
- Establish individual accounts for each person, predicating benefits on individual contributions (similar to a pension).
- Change cost-of-living adjustments (COLAs).

Benefits are currently indexed to the Consumer Price Index (CPI).

- Reduce benefits (presumably on the basis that current benefits amount to a promise that can't be fulfilled).
- Increase the amount of earnings subject to the payroll tax (currently the earned income on which payroll tax rates apply is "up to" $68,400 [1998] and there are automatic increases each year thereafter by the calculated increase in national average earnings).
- Reduce benefits for high-income beneficiaries (thus making the pay-out, or benefit function, of Social Security progressive).
- Tax Social Security like a private pension. (Employer pensions are taxed on every dollar in excess of a worker's contributions.)

In forums and town meetings, "Americans Discuss Social Security" calculates the income or loss-of-income to the trust fund of each mixture participants try to agree on. In this fashion, participants can see the sway of political opinion and how the fund can be put at risk if changes are too swift or are geared unequally to diverse age groups. Participants have to work their way through problems that affect all of society, not just the elderly or the young.

It is possible, of course, that congressional leaders will just leave Social Security alone, either because solvency is not the issue it was once thought to be, or because they will not be able to agree on drastic changes until they are forced to do so.

To appreciate the roller coaster aspect of the debate on Social Security when, understandably, the data and facts on which the debate is based changes almost daily, one need only consult

Average Monthly Benefits (Dec., 1999)	
Retired workers	$804
Aged widows (not disabled)	$775
Disabled workers	$754
Source: Social Security Administration	

news headlines in the election year 1999-2000:

- "Clinton Sparks Arguments Over Social Security Plan" (Associated Press, January 10, 1999)
- "Personal Accounts Key To Social Security Conflict" (*Aging Today*, January/February, 1999)
- "Social Security Debate Brings Out Big Money Campaigns" (Nando Media, March 10, 1999)
- "Social Security Surplus Big Boon for Economy" (*Sacramento Bee*, March 14, 1999)
- "Signs Point to Gridlock on Social Security, Medi care" (Associated Press, March 15, 1999)
- "Social Security Reform Pared Down" (Nando Media, April 17, 1999)
- "Lott Declares Social Security An Issue for Next Year" (Nando Media, April 25, 1999)
- "Social Security Changes Unlikely" (*Aging Today*, May/June, 1999)
- "What Does Fixing Social Security Actually Fix?;" "The Implications of Social Security's Long-Range Financial Projections" (Part of a series of essays published by the Urban Institute, August

19, 1999)
- "Social Security in Spotlight Again" (*Sacramento Bee*, November 6, 1999)
- "A Challenge, Not A Crisis: Forget the Election-eering Blather; We Don't Have to Upend Social Security to Save It" (*Newsweek*, July 3, 2000)

The debate seems endless, but the impacts of legislative disagreements or agreements can be very real to all Americans.

The public basis of support for Social Security is more solid today than ever. The *perception* of insolvency is more troublesome than the possibility. Former Secretary of Commerce Pete Peterson reported in his book, *Will America Grow Up Before It Grows Old?* that more young people believe in UFOs (46 percent) than think they will ever receive Social Security (28 percent) [source: Third Millennium, 1994].

In 1999, the Social Security Administration published, through its regional public affairs offices, its own assessment of "The *SIX* points to emphasize in discussions on SSA reform."

1. Social Security has made an enormous difference in the lives of Americans. ("Social Security has helped cut the poverty rate among the elderly by two-thirds—from 35% to less than 11%.")
2. Social Security is more than a retirement program ("…it is America's family protection plan, as one in three beneficiaries is not a retiree…the program's disability and survivors protection [are] invaluable…").

3. Social Security forms a solid foundation on which people can build retirement security. ("Pension and private savings have been, and are, important...but coverage is limited....")

4. Changing demographics are driving the need for change. ("Currently there are 35 million Americans age 65 and older; by 2030, there will be twice that number.")

5. People need to understand the economic facts about Social Security. It is a social insurance program. ("People who are working contribute a share of their earnings to help support those that are retired or disabled.")

6. Tough choices lie ahead of us. ("There is no perfect option...each involves difficult trade-offs....")

A 1997 study by AARP projected that outgo from the Social Security Trust Fund would substantially outstrip income by almost 2-1 by 2074. Since 1997, given the growth of the economy in the latter part of the 90s, those projections have become outdated and the "crisis" is not imminent. But even under President Clinton's announcements, there is still a date certain when solvency will be in jeopardy.

On June 7, 1998, in the "Outlook" section of *The Washington Post*, two senators and two congressmen, who are the national co-chairs of the National Commission on Retirement Policy, charted the Commission's views on change in the investment of SSA Trust funds:

Current System: Today's workers pay the bill for today's retirees through a 12.4 percent payroll tax, split evenly with employers. All the money goes to the government, which invests it in relatively low-yielding but safe United States government bonds. Retirees receive benefits according to a formula related to the highest income years of work life.

Modest Change: Shore up the financing of the existing system by letting the government invest Social Security funds in equities as well as federal instruments, increasing income taxes on Social Security benefits, raising Social Security payroll taxes in the future, and slightly cutting some benefits for future retirees.

Intermediate Change: A mixture of the old and the new: A small percentage of payroll taxes would be directed into private investments by those choosing to do so, or, in some proposals, by everyone. The remainder of the money would be allocated to the conventional Social Security program. Individuals could manage their own accounts, but some propose that the government do it. Some would increase the payroll tax for those participating in private investment.

Radical Change: This would change the Social Security system to individual investment accounts, like 401(k) plans. Employees could direct a large percentage or all of the payroll tax into private investment accounts managed by them and available to them upon retirement, passing at death to heirs. Some versions would make individual accounts mandatory for workers starting out but not for most current workers; others would allow a choice to remain in the current system.

Which of these proposals would be the best for you? Do you see a difference between a "bull" and a "bear" investment market?

Savings and Investments

Whereas Social Security is intended to provide the basics of life, people who rely on Social Security alone for their retirement income are bound to struggle to provide the necessities—and little else—for the rest of their lives.

"Most Households Not Saving Enough for Retirement, Analysis Shows," screams a headline on the front page of the Business Section of the April 27, 2000, *Los Angeles Times.* Staff writer Liz Pulliam Weston:

> "One of the most detailed retirement planning surveys to date shows that more than half of U.S. households are saving too little to maintain their current standard of living in retirement, with low-income and minority workers particularly at risk of running out of money."

The study was based on Federal Reserve statistics, the data being "...considered the most current and comprehensive information available on consumers' finances." It was sponsored by the Consumer Federation of America and Direct Advice.com, an Internet financial planning service. The actual survey was conducted by Ohio State University economics professor Catherine P. Montalto and included 2,400 households with at least one member in the work force. The major conclusion: "...only 44% of American households appear to be saving enough for retirement, based on their spending habits, retirement assets, savings rates, projected Social Security payments and expected retirement ages.

"Rather than save more, many Americans expect to live on less in retirement," the article continues. More than half (59 percent) said they would settle for less. Typically, people with higher incomes have a better chance of putting away savings or investing to meet retirement standards of living (1995 data from the AFL-CIO Public Policy Department, consistent with the Montalto study). People with lower incomes who must use more of their disposable income to live during their earning years, do not have the chance to save. The survey also found that white families are able to save or invest at almost twice the rate of black families or Latino households (47.6 percent, compared to 28.4 percent and 24.5 percent, respectively).

Pensions and Retirement Funds

At the same time, people who participate in an employer-sponsored pension plan (28 percent of the work force) are much more likely to save for retirement, regardless of race. An average of 55 percent of this group will save and invest enough for retirement. But it is also true that as income rises of participants in pension plans or employer-sponsored 401(k) plans, there is greater likelihood that higher incomes means greater savings and investment (1994 data from the AFL-CIO Public Policy Department and verified by the Montalto study).

Professor Montalto "...applied historic rates of return for each asset class—bonds, stocks, cash, home equity, real estate and business assets... the evaluation also included projected future income from Social Security [and] pension values were evaluated by estimating how much the participant was likely to receive in retirement…[her] analysis included whether the participant was a homeowner and when the mortgage was likely to be paid off…"

Perhaps the biggest culprit in not saving and investing enough for retirement is its reverse—the nation's binge on credit. Why, for example, would almost a quarter of those who are participants in an employer-sponsored pension plan NOT save enough for retirement? The plain fact is that their spending outstrips even their ability to save for their future. It may be that this is because of the cost of raising children or a strong desire to pay for an expensive education. More often, it is because of buying life's "wants" (not "needs") on credit. And, as long as families—even those with substantial incomes—are paying on never-ending debt, they will never save enough for retirement.

Which is more important? The big power boat now or the sailboat later? According to corroborating studies, the Baby Boomers have opted in greater numbers than earlier generations for the big boat now—a fact that will come home to roost for those that make that choice.

With all these warnings and admonitions, charts published by the AARP Public Policy Institute, based on 1994 data developed by Lewin-VHI, suggest that Social Security will remain the primary retirement income source in the future. In fact, AARP suggests that in 2030, 60 percent of retirement income will come from Social Security (the current percentage is 61).

Americans have much work to do if they are to forge realistic retirement plans that will meet their expectations. Who, among those who are 37 years of age today, wants to retire at 67 and rely only on Social Security?

There is statistically one exception to this scenario. It's like winning the lottery, but the odds are better. Boomers will receive the largest inheritance ever, over $10 trillion in total.

The inheritance, of course, will come from the hard work of parents who will give assets (homes, investments, and savings) to their heirs. Typically, neither parents nor heirs have prepared for this eventuality so much of the inheritance may be lost to profligate spending, mismanagement of funds, estate taxes, or court battles. Author Dan Rottenberg's *The Inheritor's Handbook: A Definitive Guide for Beneficiaries* (Bloomberg Press, 1998) may prove helpful in planning ahead.

But counting on an inheritance or the lottery is a poor gamble in retirement planning. It is far better to develop a pension plan.

Basically, there are three types of employer-sponsored pension plans, two of which usually include contributions from both the employee and the employer (contributions that can be set at any percentage for each).

A **defined benefit** plan is one in which the contribution to the plan is shared by employer and employee. But the benefit, based on a formula that is not dependent on fluctuations in the economy or investment earnings (except for the annual cost-of-living-adjustment), is constant and paid on a regular basis for the life of the retiree. The Public Employees Retirement System (PERS) of California, with more than $7 billion in assets, is the nation's most pronounced example of the defined benefit pension.

A **defined contribution** plan is one in which the contributions made by employer and employee are fixed by agreement, but the benefit, paid on a monthly or regular basis, is subject to the earnings on investments made by the plan. If the plan's earnings are up, then so are the benefits; if the earnings are down, the benefits decline correspondingly.   One of the nation's largest pension plans, TIAA-CREF, which serves college and university employees and was established by the Carnegie Foundation, is a prime example of a defined contribution plan.

A **401(k)** plan may include an employer contribution but often does not. In most cases employees "purchase" 401(k) plans with a payroll deduction. The money is invested, based on an investment option chosen by the employee, and the earnings are paid out regularly over a period of time selected by the retiree. (An IRA is similar but never includes a contribution by an employer and is usually handled entirely by the employee in choosing a financial institution and an investment option.)

The major benefit to 401(k) plans and IRAs is that the pay-out is deferred until after retirement; as a result, the income from them is taxed at the retirement income level, not the percentage of tax that applies at the time of full earning. As a result, the federal Internal Revenue code does set limits on how much of an employee's income can be invested in this manner.

Inasmuch as they are owned and managed by the employee, 401(k) portfolios and IRAs are portable; but the "defined" plans are usually restricted. PERS benefits are limited to public employees in California (including most cities, counties, and special districts). They are not portable to any other public or private employment. In the case of TIAA-CREF, plans are limited to member colleges and universities throughout the United States. They are portable among the member colleges, but not into other public or private employment.

Private employer pension plans are regulated by the Employee Retirement Income Security Act of 1974 (ERISA). For years there were horror stories about employees who had contributed to retirement plans, only to find that their employers had used the money for other purposes. Also, there were those who worked for companies that went bankrupt and found that their pensions were used to pay debts. ERISA was passed as an omnibus act on retirement and employee benefits, but primarily it guarantees employees their vested rights in retirement plans and requires companies to set aside trust funds or purchase insurance policies to back up that guarantee.

The legislative "trade-off" in exchange for the ERISA guarantee, however, is that claims against employers or insurance companies are restricted to the amount in dispute. There can be no claim for punitive damages, and bringing a claim to trial by jury is not allowed.

But pensions, even with the ERISA "guarantee," are only a part of the package. Social Security and savings and investments complete the package. With good financial planning, you should have all three.

Senior Employment
However, even if you have Social Security, savings and investments, and a pension plan, it still might not

add up to what you need in order to enhance your independence and quality of life. So you might choose part-time employment as a supplement to your income.

In today's service marketplace, employers are hiring more and more seniors. Most seniors are experienced, loyal, and reliable employees, and often they do not require benefits (many seniors already have them). Part-time employment adds to fulfillment, provides an opportunity to learn something new, and adds dollars to basic income.

In the 1970s Congress added Title V to the Older Americans Act. Title V formalized a national role in senior employment and offered recognition to employers and employees alike who emphasized the hiring and the workmanship of seniors. Title V, which today is an almost $500 million program, operates through nine major national contractors and a host of contractors in individual states and territories.

The federal appropriations are shared: 80 percent to national contractors, and 20 percent to state entities. Perhaps the three most recognized national contractors are AARP, Green Thumb, and the National Council of Senior Citizens. These contractors provide case management, along with training, job finding, and follow-up counsel to low-income "seniors" over 40, helping them to gain employment. The "low" level of 40 as a cut-off age was designed to emphasize the job-training aspect of the Title V program. Many of the contractors, like Green Thumb, specialize in the kind of work they sponsor and facilitate.

Since its inception, Title V has trained and placed tens of thousands of "seniors." When you consider that there are many low-income people who live entirely on Social Security (no savings or pensions), this element of retirement can mean that some independence and quality can be present in their lives. Without senior employment, particularly if retraining is essential, they would require institutional care, at greater expense, earlier in life.

Avoiding Scams and Fraud

It is perhaps obvious that the admonition, "Get Tough With Telemarketers" (*Modern Maturity*, AARP, by Glen Waggoner, July-August, 1999, page 79) is a caution against fraud. But the sad fact is that older adults do, in fact, need to be cautioned.

All the hard-won earnings of Social Security, savings and investments, and pension plans can be placed in jeopardy if one—just one—charlatan succeeds in sweet-talking you out of your savings. Some telemarketers will insist that they are offering a good product or good services for payment, based on your agreement to pay. Remember, they don't care a hoot about you—only your money! Beware!

Most of these scams come from telemarketers—usually sweet young voices coming over the telephone to tell you that they have a "deal for you" that is too good to be true (and it usually is).

Again, beware! Telemarketing today is a $260 billion-a-year industry! It's not all bad, but what is today's more persistent minor annoyance can be a major fraud. A simple telephone call can be an instrument of consumer fraud.

Do you know that if you request that the telemarketer STOP calling when told to do so, you have the law on your side?

Do you know that, by law, telemarketers are NOT permitted to call between 9:00 P.M. and 8:00 A.M.? "The business that doesn't honor your request to stop calling is the enemy!"

Follow some simple rules:

- Ask telemarketers for their company name and address.
- Ask about the company's refund policies.
- Ask the caller to send you written material about the company.
- Talk to advisors you trust (family, friends) before you make any large purchase or investments.
- Don't pay any fees for a prize, or send any money to improve your chances of winning "prize money."
- Never allow a caller to intimidate or bully you.
- Never give your credit card, bank account, or Social Security number to anyone over the phone, unless *you* made the call.
- Ask that your telephone number be removed from the telemarketer's list if you don't want to be called again.
- Report suspicious telemarketing calls to the state attorney general (who has jurisdiction, in most states, over the enforcement of laws regulating solicitation).

The very first line of defense against fraud is you. Make no mistake, all the official agencies in the world, and all the nonprofit do-gooders, pale by comparison, if *you* determine to be vigilant. You have worked too hard all your life to let a scam artist take away your retirement, your quality of life, and your independence.

For More Information...

Publications from **The Social Security Administration**:
Social Security Retirement Benefits (#05-10035)
Social Security–
Understanding The Benefits (#05-10024)
Call (toll free): 800-772-1213

National Committee to Preserve Social Security and Medicare
10 G Street, N.E., Suite 600
Washington, D.C. 20002-4215
202-216-0420. Hotline: 800-998-0180

Certified Financial Planner Board of Standards
1700 Broadway, Suite 2100
Denver, CO 80290-2101
303-830-7500
E-mail: mail@CFP-Board.org

U.S. Department of Labor (Senior Employment)
National Office of Public Affairs
200 Constitution Avenue, N.W.
Washington, D.C. 20210
202-693-4650

BEYOND INDEPENDENCE: INSTITUTIONAL CARE

Assisted Living and Long-term Care

Residential Care (Board and Care Homes)

Residential care is the least level of care outside the home. When independent living is no longer possible, either physically or mentally, the first—and least expensive—place to go is residential care.

Laws and regulations on residential care (also known as "Board and Care") vary from state to state, but the general standard most often reflected in the law is that residential care involves no more than six residents. Residential care facilities are usually in people's homes that have been enlarged and converted for minimal board and care. The advantage to this method of care is that it is homelike; after all, it is the home of the operator/caregiver.

If clients/patients can pay using their own resources, including some costs covered by health insurance, the state is not involved in funding. But residential care is generally designed for people with low incomes. In those cases, the state pays a daily rate, often barely meeting the actual costs. Most operators of residential care facilities have lived and worked in their communities for a lifetime and are usually well-known by neighbors. The residents, therefore, may enjoy some of the camaraderie of the neighborhood—something not available in a nursing home. Neighbors will often be mindful of residents walking in the neighborhood.

Residential care does not include medical care, but usually, health care professionals are on-call. In addition, residents may be taken to their own doctors for regular visits. In fact, residential care is considered a social service; as a result, it is regulated and inspected by social service agencies.

Assisted Living

Assisted living is a generic term referring to someone who requires assistance in performing one or more daily living tasks; hence, the term *assisted daily living* (ADL). In this context, daily living tasks include eating, dressing, bathing, going to the bathroom, etc.—tasks essential to normal physical functions in a given day. Thus, if a person has ADL needs, he or she *may* live in an assisted living facility.

It used to be that assisted living meant a nursing home, but today private corporations are building what they call "assisted living facilities" all over the United States. Thus, assisted living has taken on the meaning of a facility that is beyond residential care and short of skilled nursing care.

The first to think of a continuum of care were church-sponsored groups on the East Coast. They developed the notion that, to serve the client/patient well, retirement, assisted living, and skilled nursing should be available on one "campus." Today, these combination continuums exist nationwide.

When nursing home occupancy rates began to decline (as measured in 1995 by the CDC Nursing Home Survey), while the proportion of our population over 65 was growing, forward-thinking operators began to plan for "assisted living." Their aim was to respond to those who need a minimal level of health care, but do not require 24-hour skilled nursing care.

Thus, assisted living does include modest nursing care. A physician who agrees to be the "physician-of-record" for the facility is on-call.

Finally, assisted living facilities are often adjacent to what are colloquially known as retirement homes; that is, homes with small apartments, regular dining areas, lobbies, gardens, often a swimming pool, and libraries, along with a host of scheduled activities and trips to match the interests of just about anyone.

Long-term Care (Skilled Nursing Facilities)

Skilled nursing is required when conditions or diseases are so severe that 24-hour vigilance is required—and by a trained staff that can administer prescription drugs, monitor vital signs, and respond to emergencies.

The skill level of the professional staff is higher than that of assisted living, and not unlike the nursing staff of a hospital. Thus, patients and their families are assured that issues like pain will be addressed and that there will be regular schedules for daily functions of the body.

The nation's skilled nursing facilities ("nursing homes," although most people in the industry don't like that term) are both profit-making and not-for-profit. According to the 1995 Nursing Home Survey, two-thirds of all nursing homes in the United States are for-profit operations. More than half (55 percent) of those that are for-profit belong to large chain corporations, up from 41 percent ten years earlier. Also, since 1985, the number of all nursing homes (for-profit, nonprofit, and government-owned) decreased by 13 percent, yet the total number of beds increased by 9 percent. Thus, the trend was away from smaller homes operated by local owners and toward larger facilities that operate on economies of scale.

During the same period, there was a 23 percent drop in the number of proprietary (for-profit) homes, yet a 3 percent increase in the number of beds, meaning that large chain operations were buying out and replacing smaller homes. Ironically, however, the biggest drop in occupancy rates, according to the 1995 survey, was in the proprietary homes (85.9 percent of the previous period, lower than the average by 1.5 percent). There are some indications, as yet not surveyed, that chain operations are diminishing as a percentage of the whole. Certainly, a for-profit chain cannot sustain increasing its bed capacity by buying up competitors while they are, at the same time, experiencing the biggest drop in occupancy rates. That situation adversely impacts the "bottom line," often causing a sell-off to another chain.

In 1995, there were 1.5 million residents in the nation's 16,700 nursing homes, where more than 1.3 million full-time-equivalent (FTE) employees were working. More than one million of these employees were providing nursing services. According to Donna Shalala, former secretary of the U.S. Department of Health and Human Services, "Nursing homes remain a critical component of health care in this country and are essential to those who need intensive, 24-hour medical care. Wherever care is provided, we must ensure that it is appropriate and high quality."

Shalala's comments on quality were prompted by periodic media headlines highlighting a lack of quality in nursing home care. Some stories focused on unexplained deaths and incidents of neglect and elder abuse. When such stories appear, the reader's emotional identification with the elderly patient is instant, and the condemnation of nursing homes is strong—never enough for consumer advocates, but too much for nursing home administrators who tell us how difficult it is to operate a nursing home.

Nonprofit nursing homes seem less of a target for investigators or the media. This doesn't mean that all is well in nonprofit homes. But many nonprofits are sponsored by religious denominations and maintain a sense of spirituality about the care they provide, even if the bottom line suffers.

This doesn't mean that the for-profit operators don't care; it *does* mean that for non-profits, demonstrated caregiving is likely to be a stronger criteria in hiring staff. There are limits, however, to the ability of religious denominations to financially support skilled nursing facilities with capital, which large corporations can raise through investment. Thus, nonprofits constitute the smaller share of skilled nursing facilities.

Skilled nursing facilities also include government-owned operations, such as veterans' homes. Here all the costs are paid for by a combination of state and federal governments. Often, in the case of government facilities, budgets and staffing standards have been widely criticized.

In all these types of nursing homes, there must be licenses and inspections (oversight). This is one area in which the government is "Big Brother," and most consumers and their families would have it no other way. Nursing home operators are regulated by health departments staffed by health care professionals, many of whom have worked in and around the nursing home industry for many years. The granting of a license by the state on behalf of taxpayers and consumers is a major responsibility, which also carries with it the responsibility to make sure that the full conditions of the license are continuously met.

According to some consumer groups, many states have inadequate laws providing for sanctions against errant nursing homes. Either the fines are too small (a cost of doing business, some say), or there are procedures that the nursing home administrators, along with their lawyers, can use to reduce the tough-sounding fines to minimal amounts.

Several states have tried to enact nursing home reforms; some have been successful. But, clearly, reform movements bring on the opposition of the industry, and both sides usually complain that government reimbursement rates are not adequate. The thesis goes that the very same government that regulates nursing homes is also the provider of operating funds. If the funds are not adequate, they say, how can the same government punish (fine) them when the infractions in question are caused by insufficient funds. So it has gone, around and around, since skilled nursing facilities came into existence.

The Ombudsman Program, established by the Older Americans Act, provides an added benefit for nursing home consumers and their families. Independent of bureaucracy and composed of trained volunteers with administrative staff, ombudsmen have reasonable access to nursing homes, both to be advocates for, as well as companions to, patients and to act as watchdogs against abuse and neglect.

The privacy of the ombudsmen's investigations and reports is protected by law, and they answer only to their own administrators and courts of law, when necessary. They also witness signatures on durable Power of Attorney for Health Care forms. Ombudsmen are extra sets of eyes and ears, and their observations are the basis for larger investigations and sanctions. The "check and balance" that ombudsmen provide is essential to consumer confidence. Throughout the nation, there are more than 10,000 ombudsmen volunteers. Free training classes are held frequently. If you're interested in volunteering, your local Area Agency on Aging can help.

The Eden Alternative and Nursing Home Design

Whatever may be wrong with nursing homes today can be fixed with what William H. Thomas, M.D. says is an emphasis on values, not cost. Thomas is the author of *Life Worth Living: How Someone You Love Can Still Enjoy Life in a Nursing Home* (VanderWyk & Burnham, Acton, MA, 1996) and the founder of a reform movement called "The Eden Alternative."

Thomas doesn't diminish the issue of costs, but he rails at the bare walls of institutional care and the lack of a home atmosphere and individual expression for patients. These characteristics are avoidable, he claims, and they demean the individual when, for so little cost, life in a nursing home can be made more "homelike." All it takes, he suggests, is a modest investment, some trained volunteers, and an enlightened staff, along with some cooperative regulators.

Early in his career, Thomas never imagined himself as a nursing home doctor. But when change was needed, he allowed a friend to talk him into a "physician-of-record" post at Chase Memorial Nursing Home in New Berlin, New York. There he experienced a metamorphosis that led him to a world stage for "radical" nursing home reform.

His approach seems radical only because many nursing homes are run for the convenience of staff more than patients, and institutionalization is seen as necessary to "make the trains run on time." But what the Eden Alternative advocates is "…prescribing to residents such practical applications as companion animals and opportunities for indoor or outdoor gardening in order to create settings [that] are warm, smart and green" (*Aging*

Today, May/June, 2000, Page 5). [1] Thomas calls for "vibrant, vigorous habitats" in nursing homes.

When Thomas started his alternative movement, he ran into predictable staff resistance and rejections from public health regulators. But his is a story of persistence through the political and bureaucratic systems of the State of New York. With the fervor of a consumer advocate, the determination of his oath as a physician, and a release of energy that overwhelmed him, he overcame every hurdle. He received the various approvals he needed, and even won a grant from the State Public Health Department to try his alternative in just one nursing home. Patiently, he persuaded the staff and got them to agree to some changes. Then the resident-patients, some of whom were skeptical, also became convinced. Soon there were plants and animals in the home, and Eden was the talk of Chase Memorial. Patients and their families began to understand how much gardening meant and what the unconditional love of an animal could bring in the course of an average day.

Thomas' book tells those who will listen how to bring about such an atmosphere. The Associated Press book review said, "The book explains the Eden philosophy and provides a blueprint for putting it into action, from reorganization of staff into teams right down to the recommended type of cat litter."

The real secret? Not just birds, dogs, and cats, and not just window gardens—but staff change. The key to Eden is the staff and the empowerment of staff to be part of the decisions, including how to "Eden-ize" the home. It's not the money or even the time, but the understanding of an administrator about building teams

[1] Reprinted with permission from *Aging Today*, newspaper of the American Society on Aging, 21:3, May/June 2000, pp. 5 & 12. Copyright © 2000, American Society on Aging, San Francisco, California. www.asaging.org

and giving up top-down authority. It's not about institutions; it's about people—people with experiences and emotions, with needs and wants, with relatives and relationships, with hearts and minds. People like us.

Even before the Eden Alternative, there was a seminal study done by architect and gerontologist Victor A. Regnier, FAIA. Professor Regnier holds a unique joint appointment between the Andrus Gerontology Center and the School of Architecture at the University of Southern California. His book, *Assisted Living Housing for the Elderly: Design Innovations from the United States and Europe* (John A. Wiley & Sons, Inc., New York, 1994) includes themes for making nursing homes "...more attractive, supportive and therapeutically effective for older residents." His book, therefore, is as much about people in the settings he observes (and some that he imagines) as it is about the settings themselves. [2]

In his conclusions, he sets forth some of the practices he saw and the philosophies of management that "...make a difference..." in the lives of the residents/patients. Some of those are:

- Equity and accessibility to all income levels,
- Commitment to maintain the older person in a residential rather than an institutional environment until death,
- Supportive housing provided as part of a service continuum where resident needs and preferences dictate placement decisions,
- Community services that support the needs of family and informal caregivers,
- Project concepts that challenge conventional assumptions and existing models,

---

[2] *Assisted Living Housing for the Elderly: Design Innovations from the United States and Europe* by Victor A. Regnier, FAIA. Copyright © 1994 by Victor A. Regnier. Reprinted by permission of John Wiley & Sons, Inc.

- Rules, regulations, and standards explicit enough to ensure quality but flexible enough to encourage innovation, and
- Rural and small-town models that address individual community needs and circumstances.

There were five major issues of importance to Regnier in comparing nursing homes in northern Europe and the United States:

- Northern Europeans have designed a system that combines community services with housing for the frail, including services for older adults in the surrounding community.
- Northern Europeans use nurses and service workers to encourage even frail residents to do some things for themselves; therapeutic services build and maintain resident competency.
- They deliver "...health and personal care services to older people in a normal residential environment...including residential qualities of privacy, autonomy, personalization, and control and choice, with the concept of safety and oversight provided by the institution."
- There is respect for the professional caregiver; "in the U.S., we have created a long-term care system that is fear-based. It assumes that incompetency and violations of standards are the norm rather than recognizing professionalism and reinforcing it."
- Most new European housing models are overseen by systems regulations that encourage innovation, experimentation, and cost containment.

Hospice Services

Hospice provides services and care at home or in a facility for terminally ill patients and their families. Care is usually supervised by the family's physician, working with a team of professionals that may include nurses, social workers, the clergy, and home health care aides.

Hospice services are increasing in significance and recognized importance in the United States. The concept of community assistance to the dying is as old as mankind, but the availability of that assistance wasn't in wide use until Congress decided to provide reimbursement for the service (Medicare Hospice Benefit of 1984). With funding, the practice grew to the point where most communities now have hospice services in some form.

Hospice care primarily manages pain and discomfort while creating an environment that encourages the individual as well as loved ones to openly grieve, talk, grow, and enjoy each other while remaining physically and emotionally close until the very end. People do not usually enter hospice care until their projected final six months of life.

The National Hospice Organization estimates that more than 2,500 hospices exist in the United States today. They serve more than 300,000 people per year.

For more information on hospice locations and services, contact:

**The National Hospice and
Palliative Care Organization**
1700 Diagonal Road, Suite 300
Alexandria, VA 22314
703-837-1500
E-mail: Info@nhpco.org

For More Information...

Assisted Living Federation of America
10300 Eaton Place, Suite #400
Fairfax, VA 22030
703-691-8100
web site: www.alfa.org

American Health Care Association (ACHA)
1201 L Street, N.W.
Washington, DC 20005
202-842-4444
web site: www.ahca.org

For specific data on California nursing homes:
**California Advocates for Nursing Home Reform
(CANHR)**
1610 Bush Street
San Francisco, CA 94109
415-474-5171 or
800-474-1116 (consumer requests only)
web site: www.canhr.org

**American Association of Homes and
Services for the Aging**
901 E Street, N.W., Suite #500
Washington, DC 20004-2011
202-783-2242
E-mail: info@aahsa.org

Continued...

Eden Alternative
RD1 Box 31B4
Sherburne, NY 13460
607-674-5232
E-mail: rumpelst@norwich.net

Professor Victor A. Regnier, FAIA
School of Architecture
University of Southern California
3620 South Vermont Avenue
Los Angeles, CA 90089-2538
213-740-1357
E-mail: regnier@usc.edu

Endnote

THE BOOMERS ARE HERE —ARE WE PREPARED?

Issues That Need to Be Addressed

Baby Boomers, those born between 1946 and 1964, number 78 million Americans, the oldest of whom turned 55 in 2000. This explosion is what causes demographers to predict that between 1995 and 2020 the number of people 65 and older will double nationwide, and more than double in retirement havens like Florida, California, and Arizona.

Statistically, Boomers switch jobs, careers, even spouses, more than their parents, searching for some of the spirituality that they caught a glimpse of in their youth. For some, spirituality became conventional religion when Boomers realized that their ideas were not always transferable to their children, so the compromise was old-fashioned trips to traditional places of worship.

Thanks to their parents, Boomers are better educated than any previous generation. They are richer by far (and more pleased with their standard of living), and they stand to inherit tremendous wealth from the investments their

> ## *"The Survey Said..."*
>
> - 69% of Boomers are satisfied with their standard of living,
> - 39% of Boomer households made $60,000+,
> - 92% of Boomers have assets averaging $24,800, yet 60% say they are not saving enough to retire.
>
> —Heinz/Newsweek Poll, 4/3/00

parents made in homes and an expanding stock market. If they are able to retain this wealth, they won't have to rely only on Social Security or limited pensions.

The healthy U.S. economy of the 1990s provided Boomers with options for retirement their parents never had. But gerontologist and author Ken Dychtwald claims that many Boomers "...will age rebelliously," preferring to retire early to freelance and work part time, perhaps starting their own companies. In many ways, he argues in his book, *Age Wave* (originally published by J.P. Tarcher, Inc., Los Angeles, in 1988, and later by Bantam Books, New York), Boomers are a backlash from their parents, who were raised in the very different era of the Depression and World War II (yet these are the same parents from whom they will inherit). Their parents adopted conservative, conformist, and group-oriented lifestyles out of fear; Boomers went for the liberal, nonconformist unknown while raising the political consciousness of an entire nation to challenge what is wrong.

Other analysts and authors have puzzled endlessly over the seeming dichotomy of Boomers being pictured as rebels in younger life and materialists as they age. There seems a national penchant for describing Boomers as having evolved from idealistic, if misguided, protesters—through marriage and becoming parents—to the practical world of having to provide for themselves and the families they create. Even humorous articles, sometimes written by Boomers themselves, depict this process with a "told-you-so" flavor. More important is whether this process has delayed maturity.

What should be understood is that Boomers have established their preference for individual choice, whether in the politics of their youth or the materials with which they surround themselves now. The implication of this, of course, is that Boomers, when they become older, will continue to insist on their independence as their preferred quality of life. Accepting authority from others is anathema to many Boomers.

Questions Re Boomers

- Will the materialism of the Boomers' wage-earning years give way to a more aesthetic age of community purpose?
- Because Boomers have developed patterns of personal acquisition, will they be able to shift to themes of common interaction?

And how long will this go on? At age 55, men will live an average of 27 more years (to 82); women an average of 31 years (to 86). And, according to a survey by the Employee Benefit Research Institute, 68 percent of the people who are currently working plan to work at other jobs after they retire. The Boomers, will be around for a long time.

Social Security and Medicare

The Social Security Trust Fund is composed of employee-employer contributions, but the assets in the fund do not build, partially because for years politicians have used trust fund surpluses to fund other, often extraneous, functions of government.

By design, the current work force contributes to the fund to pay for current retirees' benefits. But now there is some fear that the work force, which is dwindling by comparison to the growing proportion of our older population, won't be able to pay the tab. On the other hand, the economy of the 1990s has produced such largesse that contributions are rolling in. Former President Clinton even announced in 2000 that, if nothing changes, the Fund will be solvent until 2063. More recent estimates place the "solvency" date at 2039, hardly an imminent crisis.

Of course, circumstances may change, causing optimism to fade. No one really knows what the impact will be on Social Security's solvency if any of the various proposals to allow a portion of retirement funds to be invested in the stock market are approved.

These proposals seemed very tempting in the 1990s, when the stock market was on a sustained roll. But, in a recession, the earnings from investments in the stock market can recoil. Some of the same people who are eager for the chance to use part of an individual Social Security account for private investment might scream "foul" in the future if they get less than what they expect. Will Congress give them a bailout, using money from the General Fund (income taxes)?

The Social Security Fund itself will suffer a downturn in a bad economy. That's why some economists and members of Congress have proposed taking Social Security "off-budget." It is "reported" now as a separate fund, but really taking it "off-budget" would mean that contributions to Social Security would stay in the trust fund and couldn't be used for other government programs. In this debate over the years, members of Congress and the Senate have been unwilling to hold Social Security sacrosanct because they have become accustomed to huge spending. Yet it stands to reason that both major parties should want the Social Security Fund "off-budget." For Republicans, it would represent a level of fiscal control not previously evident, and it would protect the covenant that Social Security represents to retirees. For Democrats, going "off-budget" would mean that the fund needs only to collect what it pays out; thus, holding out the promise of reducing payroll taxes.

Medicare, on the other hand, may have more immediate solvency issues; but even Medicare has a "witching" date in the 2020s. What may put strain on that date is the prospect that Congress and the president will agree to add prescription benefits to the program. Former President Clinton's program was more costly than congressional proposals, but both are expensive. Both parties seem to agree, however, that the high cost of prescription drugs is a serious matter requiring subsidies for seniors and the elderly. According to testimony, low-income seniors often have to choose between buying their medications or buying food!

Any action by Congress, or any downturn in the economy, will impact both Social Security and Medicare. There is no surprise in that. But it is not a crisis, as some would have you believe. As has been done many times before, congressional and executive branch leaders close ranks to keep these programs solvent when the situation—and political self-interest—demand.

Reauthorization of the Older Americans Act

With self-congratulations all around, Congress finally reauthorized the Older Americans Act, with only two dissenting votes in the House of Representatives, in October, 2000, just days before the presidential election. Never mind that reauthorization was six years overdue.

By removing contentious issues and adding a much-needed and politically attractive Family Caregiver Support Services Program (authorized and appropriated at $125 million), House and Senate members, along with contending parties among national organizations representing seniors and the elderly, set aside years of debate—and sometimes rancor—to achieve a result.

But, for six years, the lack of congressional reauthorization of Claude Pepper's seminal masterpiece was a matter of shame for those charged with the trust of the Act. There was plenty enough blame to go around, and there were excuses—but there were no adequate reasons. Not only was the reauthorization overdue—the Older Americans Act is usually updated every five years—it was on its second cycle of being overdue.

For six years, while Congress was guilty of benign neglect and sending a discouraging signal to the "aging network," money *did* continue to flow into OAA programs. But that money lost 40 percent of its purchasing power. In Congress, the authorization of policymaking legislation contains target dollar figures, but congressional rules require that appropriations be enacted in budget bills in order for funds to be delivered. Thus, the Area Agencies on Aging operate on previously established policy, even if it is not updated, as long as Congress appropriates money. Logically, Congress should set the policy (authorization) first and then appropriate to meet the policy. But, in the case of OAA, Congress continued to appropriate on the basis of policy that was eleven years old.

How can this be? It was because of squabbling on two major items—the national funding formula and senior employment (Title V). The funding formula issue is a traditional battle between urban, suburban, and rural states. In the final reauthorization, it was politically easier to make only minor changes in the formula, retaining essentially the same proportions as were negotiated eleven years earlier.

But that's only a political resolution. In reality, there were major population shifts during those years, and the formula should have been updated to reflect those changes. Once the matter is on the table, however, each state attempts to carve the best deal for itself. As with any funding formula, whether it's social services or transportation or military spending, compromise is necessary to reach enactment—but a major compromise apparently wasn't possible, so the bill's authors fell back on only minor changes.

Instead, Congress crafted the Caregivers Program, which has the effect of earmarking for support of caregivers money that probably should have been appropriated, but wasn't, during the delay in reauthorization. This is not to say that caregiver support services aren't important; it is, however, a politically expedient way to wrap what should have been done all along in an appealing package.

Perhaps more a cause of the delay was Title V, which funds employment training and placement for seniors. Early in the Clinton Administration it was proposed that the management of Title V be transferred from the Department of Labor to the Administration on Aging. At the same time, the Administration proposed that some of the dollars awarded to national contractors be shifted to state contractors. The incumbent national contractors claimed that such changes risked destroying a good program.

To put the matter in perspective, it should be understood that Title V has grown to almost $500 million, and 80 percent of that, by law, goes to national contractors, of which there are nine. Three of the major contractors are AARP, the National Council of Senior Citizens, and Green Thumb. (Green Thumb's total income is derived from Title V.) Inasmuch as 10 percent of the contract funds (or $36 million at the national level) are allowed for administrative costs, it was clear that incumbent national contractors wanted nothing changed. One of them even contacted its members nationwide to ask them to lobby against the reauthorization of OAA unless Title V was left intact.

That successful lobbying effort did not go unnoticed for its irony. Here was a prominent organization ostensibly providing a service for seniors fiercely lobbying against the reauthorization of an omnibus bill benefiting seniors.

With President Clinton's signature, this frustrating saga came to a close. Certainly, some result was better than continued neglect. But the clock is ticking on the next reauthorization already. By the end of the year 2005, there should be a new reauthorization with an updated policy, including funding formulas and changes in Title V.

Resources (Federal, State, and Local)

The exponential growth in the number of seniors and frail elderly will place an ever-increasing demand on the services provided by the Older Americans Act. And Congress will have to step up to the plate each year!

Only once, in 1998, were federal funds for OAA increased. Then-Senator Al D'Amato (R-NY) championed an increase of more than $20 million in Title III (congregate and in-home delivered meals). His move was unexpected but gratefully received by the "aging network" that had been ignored on funding increases for years, in spite of increased demand.

In context, however, federal funding for OAA has lost much of its purchasing power, especially in programs providing meals and transportation. The major exception to this pattern is the home health industry, which serves many of the same seniors and frail elderly served by OAA. The home health industry has grown dramatically in recent years, along with the appropriations that support it. In the main, however, routine appropriations for OAA reflected the congressional demeanor on reauthorization.

What may cause alarm within the "network," however, is the advent of the Baby Boomers. The number of people 65 and over is already growing exponentially. "Network" service administrators and providers know this, and they want to prepare for the future demand. Legislators, however, often react instead of act, and so it seems that, for now, they will await a popular expression on aging issues before reacting.

Meanwhile, the states seem to be more energetic, if only because state legislators are closer to an increasing demand and want to be counted as supportive of individual state versions of the OAA. Also, the most recent Nursing Home Survey, conducted by the Centers for Disease Control and Prevention, showed that occupancy rates in nursing homes are declining for the first time in history. That fact played a major role in convincing legislators that investment in social programs for older adults was enabling those adults to live independently longer.

Moreover, at the state level there has been considerable focus on the integration of services. The goal of integration is to provide easy access to services (from toll-free telephone numbers to effective case management) and to organize a continuum of care that is flexible enough to meet changes in consumer choice and in physical or mental conditions. The continuum crosses the boundaries separating health and social services (often carefully guarded bureaucratic turf) to offer the combination of services needed by the consumer/patient. The focus of this effort is the person receiving the services, not the institutional provider.

The result of these concerns is awareness at the state level that seems to be reflected in considerable increases in funding. California, for example, has had two recent budget increases in its Older Californians Act programs after nine years of a "dry spell." And those increases came in the last year of a Republican Administration and the first year of the successor Democratic one. State-level increases seem to be bipartisan, while service integration takes executive branch leadership to bridge bureaucratic gaps. In New Jersey, for example, then-Governor Christie Todd Whitman issued an executive order forcing integration to take place.

At the local level, the gap between supply and demand has been addressed with the advent of thousands of volunteers. Current estimates suggest that there are between 650,000 and 700,000 volunteers supporting the programs of the Older Americans Act and state companion acts. The value of these services is greater than federal and state appropriations combined.

Outreach Programs

It is a nagging dilemma for social service planners—programs exist, sometimes in abundance, but people don't know about them. Simply stated, that is a function of outreach—literally reaching out through advertising (television, radio, printed brochures, mailers, etc.)

and community word-of-mouth—to make sure that those who could use these services *know* that they have the choice.

Budget planners, on the other hand, worry that too much outreach will result in greater utilization of programs, which will increase costs. Within government, this is a major tug-and-pull. But recently, it has been shown that social services help to increase the chance that the elderly remain as independent as possible for as long as possible. The Nursing Home Survey by the Centers for Disease Control shows a decrease in nursing home occupancy rates. Experts attribute this decline to the increase in home health care services, new medical technologies and home- and community-based services.

Thus, social services are a good investment when contrasted with institutional care, even if there is greater demand on social programs because of an increase in the older population and better efforts at outreach. Another way to look at this policy-and-budget dilemma is to ask what the costs might be if we didn't have these social services and if we didn't extend them to those in need.

Family Caregiving

In 1998, the U.S. Senate Special Committee on Aging held a hearing on "family caregiving." The keynote witness was former First Lady Rosalynn Carter, and the essence of her testimony was:

> With exponentially advancing numbers of older Americans, it is past due that Congress must recognize that caregiving for the elderly is as much a social responsibility as child care.

Mrs. Carter suggested, too, that many more working families will be involved in caregiving as their parents age. This, she said, is a problem for employers whose employees will, in greater numbers, have to take leave from their jobs to care for their parents, especially if there are serious health issues, physical or mental.

The addition of the Family Caregivers Support Services Program to the Older Americans Act is a clear example that members of Congress now seem to recognize the true costs of caregiving. And while there is now a provision for tax credits for caregivers, the real concern is for job security in a world where the practical demands of caregiving can take an inordinate amount of time away from jobs. With this in mind, Mrs. Carter suggested that until caregiving for an older parent or close relative is included in the guarantees of the Family Leave Act, employees will not have peace of mind. Without that peace of mind, employees will experience greater stress, which will impair their performance on the job.

The Family Leave Act is still fairly new. Statistics on the effects of this legislation are just now being calculated, so it may not be surprising that Congress has not yet embraced added coverage under the Act. But there are a number of members of Congress, Republicans and Democrats alike, who have joined Mrs. Carter in her assertion.

In the meantime, of course, there is a myriad of volunteer, nonprofit associations, with chapters throughout the nation, offering counseling and support services to those in a caregiving role. These groups, such as the Alzheimer's Association, provide a strong haven for people who may be comparatively new to caregiving. Surely, being a caregiver will be an experience almost all of us will have. How will we look at the task—as a burden, a privilege, or both? How will our attitude affect those we love? How will we be affected?

Caregiving is, first and foremost, the giving of one's self.

APPENDIX A

Diseases and Conditions
That Adversely Impact the Elderly

Accident Prevention (Falls, Mobility Disorders, and Driving)

Are accidents preventable? Of course they are. Staying in good physical and mental health so that you are alert and able to "catch yourself" is vital. More importantly, it makes sense to be safe; that is, to take common-sense steps to avoid the risks associated with accidents.

Make no mistake about it, accidents, especially those involving older adults and frail elderly, are serious matters. How many times have you heard people say about an elderly person that an accidental fall was the "trigger" for other maladies that can weaken the will to live?

Leading the categories of accidents that cause serious harm are falls, burns, and motor vehicle crashes. All are preventable!

- "Three-fourths of deaths due to falls occur in the 13 percent of the population aged 65 years and older." (Rubenstein, L.Z.; Josephson, K.R.; Robbins, A.S.; *Falls in the Nursing Home*, 1994). [1]
- "Accidents are the fifth leading cause of death among older adults and falls account for two-thirds." [2]
- "Studies have shown falls and instability to be precipitating causes of nursing home admissions." [3]
- "Older adults with lower extremity weakness have about a six-fold increase in fall risks, and persons with an impaired gait or balance have a four- and five-fold increase, respectively." [4]
- "Motor vehicle accidents are the most common cause of accidental death among the 65 to 74 age group and the second most common cause among older people in general." (National Institute on Aging, 1991 data).
- "People over age 65 make up about 12 percent of the population and suffer 27 percent of all accidental deaths." (National Institute on Aging, 1991 data).

---

[1] Reprinted in "New Facts About...Falls and Mobility Disorders in Older Adults," published jointly by RAND Corporation and Pfizer U.S. Pharmaceuticals, February, 2000. Copyright 2000 by Pfizer U.S. Pharmaceuticals. Reprinted by permission.

[2] ibid.

[3] ibid.

[4] ibid.

Older adults have more accidents simply because of the health problems of aging. Poor eyesight, loss of hearing, arthritis, neurological diseases, and problems with balance cause people to be unsteady. That's why there are canes, walkers, and wheelchairs.

Medications, too much alcohol, depression, drowsiness, and distraction—all are contributors to mishaps. In the elderly with bone loss (osteoporosis), falls can mean broken bones, from which it is hard to recover. Similarly, slower reaction thus leads to injuries and burns. Recovering from burns can be slow and painful.

This is not a time for mincing words about driving a vehicle when you are impaired. This has become a major national issue because Americans are in love with their cars, and most people, especially men, have driven throughout their teenage and adult lives.

Many—even most—older adults consider it "the beginning of the end" of life if they can't drive anymore. They can't stand the stigma, and they consider even questioning the driving ability of an older person to be insulting and discriminatory.

Yes, impairment, physical or mental, that adversely affects your ability to

---

Driving Programs

AARP 55 Alive
(Mature driver program)
1909 K Street, N.W.
Washington, D.C. 20049
800-424-3410

AAA Foundation for Traffic Safety
1730 M Street, N.W., #401
Washington, D.C. 20036
800-305-SAFE

drive can happen at any age, and most of us support a state drivers' licensing system that tests for driving ability after reaching a certain minimum age and periodically thereafter. But impairment that affects driving will inevitably occur in older adults. It's not a matter of "whether or not"—it's a matter of "when." Impairment will set in sooner in some than in others.

But it makes no sense to continue to drive, for any reason, especially if it is a matter of ego, once impairment sets in. It makes no sense to put other people on the road at risk (even if it's only a trip to the corner grocery).

Most states are in the throes of legislative debate on this issue, and most are moving toward mandatory driver testing after a certain age. Advocates for seniors argue that, because impairment can occur at any time, special age-designated testing is discriminatory. Yet, as we age, our faculties fail. There's nothing wrong or discriminatory about it; it happens to all of us. It is a normal function of aging. When the time comes, sit back, relax, and enjoy being chauffeured by family, friends, and volunteers, often at no cost to you. And lobby your state and local governments for better transit systems, more designated seating for seniors, and paratransit so that you can plan and practice using alternative forms of transport.

"An Ounce of Prevention..."

- Install light switches at the bottom and top of stairways.

- Use bedside remote-control light switches.
- Install sturdy handrails on both sides of stairways.
- Tack down carpeting or use non-skid treads on stairs.
- Remove throw rugs; trail electrical cords along walls.
- Arrange furniture to use, not as obstacles.
- Install grab bars and non-skid mats in bathrooms.
- Keep outdoor steps and walkways in good repair.
- If you do smoke, never smoke in bed.
- Don't wear loose-fitting clothing when you're cooking.
- Don't let water heater thermostats or hot faucets cause scalding.
- When lifting, bend your knees; when reaching, stretch.
- Do you know where your emergency exits are?
- Be careful with appliances, especially space heaters.
- When using public transportation, stay alert, brace yourself, be careful of slippery pavement, have your fare ready, and always have one hand free to hold on.

AIDS, HIV, and Older Adults

AIDS (Acquired Immunodeficiency Syndrome) and its precursor, HIV (Human Immunodeficiency Virus) are not limited to younger people, who are typically viewed as being sexually active. If you are sexually active at any age, HIV and AIDS should be your concern, too.

AIDS is caused by HIV, which attacks the body's immune system. When your immune system is weakened, it can't fight diseases as it does normally. Thus, HIV and AIDS are not direct causes of death, but HIV leads to AIDS, which leads to immune deficiency, which leads to pneumonia and other conditions, which lead to death. Older adults already have slightly weakened immune systems; HIV and AIDS will hurry that weakening process. Thus, an older adult may die faster of AIDS than a younger person.

This is not a pretty picture—but HIV and AIDS are preventable! HIV is spread from one infected person to another, almost entirely by sexual activity through the exchange of bodily fluids (semen, blood [not saliva] and vaginal fluids). It used to be that HIV could be contracted from blood transfusions, but intense screening since 1985 has all but eliminated transfusions as a source of HIV. And HIV *cannot* be contracted through casual contact with an infected person—not touching, coughing, sneezing, or using the same restroom or telephone.

How do you prevent AIDS? If your sexual partner is not someone you *know* to be uninfected and mutually faithful, use a condom! It's that simple. If you get HIV, how-

---

The Truth

"The truth is that 11 percent of all new AIDS cases are now in people age 50 and over.

"And in the last few years, new AIDS cases rose faster in middle-age and older people than in people under 40."

From the U.S. Administration on Aging web site, National Institute on Aging: www.aoa.dhhs.gov/aoa/pages/agepages/aids.html 1/22/00.

ever, there is treatment—usually AZT, a drug that does not cure AIDS but may let you stay healthier longer. In addition, there are major research efforts aimed at finding more effective treatments. The media reports on many of these treatments as a result of studies presented at worldwide AIDS conferences. But to date, the most often prescribed drug is AZT or a "cocktail" mixture of AZT and other drugs.

AIDS is hard to detect in older adults because its symptoms (tiredness, loss of appetite, and swollen glands) are similar to a number of other conditions and may be thought to be minor. As in other diseases and conditions, do not hesitate to consult your doctor and be prepared for your visit (see "Doctor Dialogue," Page 44).

For general information and local referrals, call the National AIDS Hotline at 800-342-AIDS (800-344-SIDA for Spanish and 800-AIDS-889 for TTY). AARP also maintains a Social Outreach and Support (SOS) unit at 202-434-2260 (601 E Street, NW, Washington, DC, 20049).

Alcohol Abuse and Alcoholism

If you think that alcohol is abused only by the young, think again. Most older alcoholics have been chronic abusers of alcohol for years. Oh, yes, there can be abusers who are "situational." These are people who, later in life, have trouble dealing with changes or crises such as illness, reduced income, loneliness, and the deaths of close friends or family. While drinking offers the illusion of relief, it can develop into a chronic problem.

Such an admonition is not meant to stem moderate drinking on social occasions. The company of friends can be enhanced by a good wine, a satisfying beer, or a fine-tasting liqueur. But such occasions are not a reason to drink to excess.

Excessive drinking has consequences that are exaggerated with age. Alcohol affects the brain; hence, alertness and coordination. This increases the risk of falls. And falling on more brittle bones can mean a hospital stay, even surgery. Also, alcohol changes blood vessels, which, in turn, can dull pain and inhibit the body's natural warning system for serious events like heart attacks. Heavy drinking over time can cause damage to the nervous system, heart, stomach, and liver. This makes other illnesses harder to diagnose.

Older people are proportionately larger users of over-the-counter and prescription drugs; and mixing alcohol with drugs can aggravate medication management issues (see "Managing Your Meds," Page 60). Adverse reactions can be fatal if alcohol is mixed with sleeping pills, painkillers, tranquilizers, or antihistamines. Take the example of simple aspirin. According to the Surgeon General, aspirin can cause bleeding in the stomach. When you combine aspirin with alcohol, the risk of internal bleeding is much higher.

The National Institute on Aging provides a list of indicators of a drinking problem. Check it against your own habits. Seek help if you:

- Drink to calm your nerves, forget your worries, or reduce depression,
- Black out or experience time loss (forgetting),
- Lose interest in food,
- Gulp your drinks down fast,

- Lie about, or try to hide, your drinking habits,
- Drink alone more often,
- Hurt yourself, or someone else, while drinking,
- Were drunk more than three or four times last year,
- Need more alcohol to get "high,"
- Feel irritable, resentful or unreasonable when you are not drinking, or
- Have medical, social, or financial problems caused by drinking.

For More Information...

The National Institute on Aging Information Center
P.O. Box 8057
Gaithersburg, MD 20898-8057
800-222-2225

The National Institute on Alcohol Abuse and Alcoholism
6000 Executive Boulevard
Bethesda, MD 20892-7003
301-443-3860

The National Council on Alcoholism and Drug Dependence
12 West 21st Street, 8th Floor
New York City, NY 10010
800-NCA-CALL (800-222-4225)

Or check your telephone book for the number of your local chapter of Alcoholics Anonymous.

Alzheimer's Disease

Is there anyone who could not identify with former President Ronald Reagan when he wrote a note informing the American people that he had Alzheimer's Disease? Few famous people admit to infirmities or conditions that might suggest weakness. President Reagan, in his characteristically straightforward manner, created a level of awareness for average Americans about a disease that was previously known mostly to those who were afflicted and their families.

In recent times, the nearest parallel to this kind of selflessness was seen in prominent women who spoke up about their own breast cancer, thus providing a "home" of understanding for the tens of thousands similarly afflicted—and their husbands and families.

Millions of words have been written about Alzheimer's; we won't attempt here to paraphrase or condense those words. We suggest that, if you have a family member with Alzheimer's and you need help, turn to the Alzheimer's Association and its hundreds of local chapters throughout the nation. There you will find kindred souls and knowledgeable people who will provide a support system.

Suffice to say that Webster's Dictionary provides only a curt definition: "a degenerative brain disease, named after a 20th century German physician, A. Alzheimer." This definition, of course, masks the detail and doesn't include the levels of research into potential medical treatment, the devotion that hundreds of thousands of people give to caregiving for loved ones, or the networks of organizations and volunteers throughout the world.

Alzheimer's is very hard to diagnose in its beginning stages. As a *Newsweek* article (January 31, 2000) said, "Forgetting the date or losing keys may not indicate the onset of Alzheimer's. But if these common traits worsen, they may form the disease's recognizable pattern." It is important for family members to understand that an autopsy can confirm the existence of Alzheimer's through the discovery of plaques on the brain, indicating the irretrievable loss of memory. Often this is the only pathway to serious research into diagnosis and treatment for others.

Research by Stephen Totilo of the Alzheimer's Association, outlined in the *Newsweek* article, identified three stages of Alzheimer's:

Early Stage
- Recent memory loss begins to affect job performance
- Confusion about places
- Loses initiative
- Mood/personality changes; avoids people
- Takes longer with routine chores
- Makes bad decisions
- Trouble with handling money, paying bills

Middle Stage
- Increasing memory loss and confusion
- Problems recognizing close friends
- Repetitive statements
- Occasional muscle twitches or jerking
- Motor problems
- Problems with reading, writing, and numbers

- Difficulty in thinking logically
- Can't find right words
- May be suspicious, irritable, fidgety, teary
- Loss of impulse control, refusal to bathe, has trouble dressing
- May see or hear things that are not there
- Needs supervision

Late Stage
- Loses weight; can't remember when they ate and how much
- Can't recognize family members or image of self in mirror
- Unable to care for self, wandering from home or care center
- Can't communicate
- May put everything in mouth, touch everything
- Can't control bowels, bladder
- May have seizures, difficulty with swallowing, skin infections

---

Mini-Mental State Examination... [5]

A test, copyrighted in 1975, was re-developed in 1998 by Mini-Mental, LLC. The test can help physicians spot a potential Alzheimer's victim. There are 30 possible points. Average scores are 29 for those with at least nine years of education and 22 for those with fewer years; the overall average is 25.

---

[5] "Mini-Mental State: A Practical Method for Grading the Cognitive State of Patients for the Clinician." *Journal of Psychiatric Research*, 12(3): 189-198, 1975. Copyright © 1975, 1998 by Mini-Mental, LLC, Boston, MA. Reprinted with permission.

Max Score	Question
	Orientation
5	What is the (year)(season)(day)(month)?
5	Where are we: (state)(county)(town) (hospital)(floor)?
	Registration
3	Name three unrelated objects. Allow one second to say each. Ask the patient to repeat all three after you have said them. Give one point for each correct answer. Repeat them until he or she learns all three.
	Attention and Calculation
5	Ask patient to count backward from 100 by sevens. Give one point for each correct answer. Stop after five.
	Recall
3	Ask patient to recall the three objects previously stated. Give one point for each correct answer.
	Language
2	Show patient a wristwatch; ask patient what it is. Repeat for a pencil.
1	Ask patient to repeat the following: "No ifs, ands, or buts."
3	Ask patient to follow a three-stage command: "Take a paper in your right hand, fold it in half, and put it on the floor."

Continued

1	Ask patient to read and obey the following sentence, which you have written on a piece of paper: "Close your eyes."
1	Ask patient to write a sentence.
1	Ask patient to copy a design.
30	**Total Possible Score**

How well would you do, knowing that you have yet to reach "forgetful?" Of course, this is not a test that is one-time-only; it should be given over time to evaluate patterns. But it can also act as a warning sign to physicians who must alert family members and caregivers. Early intervention can mean treatment, such as placement in an adult day health center (see section on "Support Programs and Services," page 123), which can vastly improve quality of life.

For more information and local referral:

The Alzheimer's Association
919 No. Michigan Avenue, Suite 1100
Chicago, IL 60611
800-272-3900
web site: www.alz.org

Alzheimer's Disease Education and Referral Center
P.O. Box 8250
Silver Spring, MD 20927
800-438-4380
E-mail: adear@alzheimers.org

Arthritis (Rheumatoid Arthritis, Osteoarthritis)

When the older adults of today visited their grand-mothers, they were likely to hear complaints about arthritis, which Edition 28 of Dorland's Medical Dictionary (1994, W.B. Saunders Company, Philadelphia) describes simply as, "the inflammation of the joints."

Arthritis is commonplace; in fact, it affects half of those over 65. Your grandmother was the rule, not the exception. While there are medications to treat arthritis (cortizone and its derivatives are used most often) and therapy to minimize pain and disability and improve joint mobility, there is no cure. In further fact, arthritis can come and go in many people; thus, giving the illusion of a cure—but the arthritis most often returns. This is why scam artists, offering for sale some magical "cure" for arthritis, often claim that their product is a true elixir for which, of course, they charge an exorbitant price.

But when your grandmother spoke of her arthritis, she meant "rheumatoid arthritis," described in Dorland's as "...a chronic systematic disease primarily of the joints...marked by inflammatory changes...and by muscle atrophy." Today, doctors have linked arthritis with osteoporosis (bone loss), mostly in women, and called it "osteoarthritis." This means that the arthritis is "degenerative" and that the "inflammation" may be more severe.

Evidence from The Framingham Osteoarthritis Study, reprinted in February, 2000, under a joint three-year collaboration between Pfizer U.S. Pharmaceuticals and The RAND Corporation, concluded that 27 percent of people 65-69, and 51 percent of those 85 and older, have osteoarthritis. It accounts for half of all disabilities among older adults.

Therapy, selective use of medications, and education about arthritis and its effects and treatments are the best weapons against the disease. Be aware, however, that some therapies carry with them some added risks, so appropriate therapy for arthritis should be specifically tailored to a patient's individual needs. In more extreme cases, surgical replacement of a knee or hip will provide "substantial improvements" in function and quality of life.

For further information on osteoarthritis or rheumatoid arthritis, contact:

The Arthritis Foundation
1330 West Peachtree Street
Atlanta, GA 30309
800-283-7800

Blood Pressure (Hypertension)

High blood pressure (HBP or hypertension) is something to watch and manage; it is not something to fear. But make no mistake, if you don't watch it, high blood pressure can lead to strokes, heart disease, kidney failure, and other health problems.

The *average* blood pressure is 120/80, usually expressed as "one-twenty over eighty." *Normal* blood pressure can range from 110 to 140. That's the "upper," or "systolic," reading. In older adults that number is likely to go higher than the average, necessitating some level of treatment, often not more than a change in diet. Lower diastolic readings are usually not something to worry about.

Keys to Prevention

- Maintain moderate weight.
- Cut down on salt.
- Exercise regularly (see "Exercise and Fitness," Page 53).
- If you drink, have no more than two drinks a day.

Most of us are familiar with blood pressure readings. Taken with an air cuff placed around your arm, the doctor or nurse pumps air into the cuff, lets the air out gradually, and takes the reading as the air escapes. The cuff is reading the pressure against blood vessel walls as blood flows from your heart outward.

Volumes of studies over decades show conclusively that bringing the systolic (upper) number down closer to the average (120) cuts down significantly on strokes and heart attacks. Measuring your blood pressure is so simple, quick, and pain-free that it makes sense to take your blood pressure often—just to give yourself a checkup.

There are even free blood pressure machines in shopping malls and pharmacies that you can operate yourself. And, if you notice that the upper number is closer to 140 than 120, see your doctor and ask him or her to measure your blood pressure professionally and suggest some simple lifestyle changes that can save you stress with absolute ease and no discomfort. It just makes common sense.

Blood pressure is a silent, but important, function of your body. You don't notice it unless you are exercising or under stress. If your blood pressure goes up during exercise, that's normal. It's when it goes up without exercise or stress that you should take note. Maybe your salt intake is too high, maybe you're overweight, or maybe you're drinking too much alcohol. Those habits increase the chance of HBP. But those are things in your life that you can change with varying effort. And remember, when you do make such changes, you are reducing your risk of a heart attack or a stroke. Isn't that worth it?

You can't cure HBP, but you can control it just by compensating for the habits that have contributed to it. If necessary, your physician can prescribe drugs that "hold" blood pressure down, but these are expensive drugs. Thus, you can be your own best friend by maintaining your blood pressure in the normal range with good habits that compensate for the causes of HBP in your own situation.

The important goal is to get into a routine of diet and medicines, if necessary, that can maintain your blood pressure close to average.

For More Information...

The National Heart, Lung and Blood Information Center
P.O. Box 30105
Bethesda, MD 20824-0105
301-251-1222

The National Institute on Aging Information Center
P.O. Box 8057
Gaithersburg, MD 20898-8057
800-222-2225

For example, the Administration on Aging advises that those who are using a prescription for high blood pressure get into the habit of taking the medicine at the same easy-to-remember time every day (perhaps when you are brushing your teeth in the morning or evening).

The Administration on Aging calls HBP "...a common but controllable disorder." But, of course, you must know about it, and you must make choices to exercise control. For your own sake, that's *your* responsibility. Read more, if you wish, by contacting AoA's web site at www.aoa.dhhs.gov/aoa/pages/agepages/hibldpr/html.

Cancer

The mere mention of cancer connotes trauma, but there are myriad stories about ordinary people who have braved the rigors of cancer treatment to live full and lengthy lives.

There's no room to be a Pollyanna. But neither is there cause to suggest that a diagnosis of cancer means the end of life or of a reasonable quality of life. There are many "survivors" of breast cancer, now organized into local support groups, who are living life to the fullest, taking reasonable precautions, and who expect to live as long as others and probably die, when their time comes, of something else. And rates of "survival" are increasing exponentially.

Yet, it is axiomatic that early detection of any kind of the over 100 types of cancer means a far better chance of successful treatment. So it makes sense for you to consult the risk factors and warning signs of the various major varieties of cancer.

Major national organizations that address all cancers are:

The American Cancer Society
1599 Clifton Road, N.E.
Atlanta, GA 30329-4251
800-ACS-2345
web site: www.cancer.org

The National Cancer Institute
9000 Rockville Pike, Bldg. 31
Bethesda, MD 20892
800-4CANCER
web site: www.cancer.gov

Breast cancer: The primary risks for breast cancer are:

- A family history of breast cancer (mother, sister, aunt)
- A previous breast cancer
- A history of breast cell abnormalities (lumpy breasts are not counted as "abnormal")
- Early menstruation (before age 12)
- Late menopause (Both early menstruation and late menopause result in greater exposure to estrogen hormones, which can increase the possibility of breast cancer)
- No children/older age for first birth—pregnancy actually enhances protection against breast cancer.

As is the case with all health conditions and diseases, there are lifestyle habits or other physical conditions that can act as secondary risks:

- Obesity,
- Lack of exercise,
- A high-fat diet (lots of red meat),
- Excess consumption of alcohol,
- Some artificial hormones (hormone replacement therapy), primarily estrogen alone,
- Environmental factor (exposure to carcinogens, such as pesticides or DDT, where there may not have been a demonstrated cause and effect, but where there is substantial epidemiological evidence of harm),
- Electromagnetic fields, such as living in proximity to power lines, and
- Radiation exposure, such as X-rays, at a young age.

Taken individually, these secondary risks mean little; taken together or in conjunction with one or more of the primary risks, the risk can be noticeable.

> ### A Clearinghouse on Breast Cancer
>
> **The National Alliance of Breast Cancer Organizations (NABCO)**
> 1180 Avenue of the Americas
> 2nd Floor
> New York, NY 10036
> 888-80NABCO
> web site: www.nabco.org

Examinations and mammography, undertaken regularly, serve as early warnings for breast cancer; therefore, routine visits with health professionals, and more frequent visits as you grow older, are strongly advised. Always remember that early detection of all types of cancer increases the chances of successful treatment or intervention.

The advisories given to women on what these routines should be have varied in recent years as medical professionals try to balance patient care against a new rise in health care costs. Almost any author now will qualify his or her advice by suggesting that the advice is under continuing review; however, one current advisory published by the National Alliance of Breast Cancer Organizations website recommends:

1. All women, from age 20, should conduct their own breast examination every month (with questions or concerns addressed to physicians).

2. Additionally, beginning at age 20, all women should have their breasts examined by a physician or nurse (a "clinical" breast examination)

3. Women, upon reaching age 40, should get a mammogram (breast X ray) each year.

Colon cancer: On colon (or colorectal) cancer we found a guide written by a patient but strongly endorsed by a body of physicians, *Colon Cancer and the Polyps Connection* by Stephen Fisher, published in 1995 by a family firm, Fisher Books. Fisher tells his highly compelling and inspirational story first; then he details the major issues concerning colon cancer so that readers can learn from what he has gleaned.

As in all cancers, the key to treatment of colon cancer is early detection. During routine physical examinations, your doctor can conduct a "digital rectal"—a polite way of describing the insertion of a gloved and lubricated finger into the anus to feel for polyps. Also, your doctor can ask you to provide a sample of your stool, usually obtained with a wooden tongue depressor and placed on a specially designed cardboard folder for evaluation in a laboratory. The doctor will be checking for the presence of blood in the stool. Then, if indicated, the doctor can conduct a sigmoidoscopy, a procedure in which a proctoscope (a tube with a small camera on the tip) is inserted up into the rectum to look for polyps, which can be clipped and biopsied in a lab to check for cancer. If cancer is discovered, then appropriate treatment can be discussed and agreed to by you and your physician.

Those who are said to be at high risk (greater than the general population) are people who have:

- A previous diagnosis of bowel cancer or polyps,
- Close relatives with the same diagnosis, especially if they are under 55,
- A previous diagnosis of numerous ulcers lining the large bowel for more than 10 years, or
- A history (women) of breast, ovarian, or endometrial cancer, or a family history of polyposis or Gardner's Syndrome (1 percent of colon cancer patients).

Those who are said to have an average risk (most people) are:

- Over 40 (55+ percent of those with colon cancer are over 40) with chances to develop colon cancer doubling each decade after age 40.

The warning signs for colon (colorectal) cancer are:

- Bleeding in the stool, or a stool that is black in color,

- Pain—gnawing abdominal pain for more than a week,
- A change in bowel habits (whatever they are for you),
- Tenesmus—an urgent, painful need to have a bowel movement, coupled with the feeling of not being able to empty the rectum,
- Narrowing of the stool, indicating digestion concerns, and
- Unexplained weight loss, intermittent gas, lack of appetite, anemia, and unusual paleness and fatigue.

Both the American Cancer Society and the National Cancer Institute, listed at the beginning of this section on cancers, are able to send you free copies of booklets on colon cancer.

Ovarian cancer: There is a blood test to detect ovarian cancer, but its reliability has been questioned. Thus, caution is advised. To be certain, assess the following list of risks and warnings published by The Ovarian Cancer Research Fund in a special educational supplement in the October 1999, issue of *Harper's Bazaar*. The supplement was a tribute to the Bazaar's Editor-in-Chief, Liz Tilberis, who had died of ovarian cancer in April. Tilberis wrote an autobiography entitled *No Time To Die*.

You are at increased risk of ovarian cancer if:
- You have a mother, sister, or daughter who has had ovarian cancer,
- You have a personal history of breast cancer or the genetic markers for breast or ovarian cancer,

- You are of Ashkenazi Jewish descent and have a genetic marker,
- You have never been pregnant, or
- You are over 60. The leading risk factor is increasing age. A woman's risk at age 40 is 15.7 per 100,000; at age 79, the risk is 54 per 100,000.

The symptoms of ovarian cancer are vague. But if one or more of the following symptoms *persist for a month*, consult your gynecologist or a gynecologic oncologist immediately:

- Vague but persistent gastrointestinal discomfort, such as gas, nausea and/or indigestion,
- A frequent or urgent need to urinate,
- A change in bowel habits,
- Abnormal vaginal bleeding,
- Pelvic or abdominal swelling that may or may not be accompanied by pain; bloating or a feeling of fullness,
- Loss of appetite and feeling full even after a light meal,
- Unexplained fatigue,
- Shortness of breath,
- Pain during intercourse, or
- Unexplained weight gain or loss.

For More Information...

The Ovarian Cancer Research Fund
1 Penn Plaza, Suite 1610
New York, NY 10119-0165
800-873-9569
web site: www.ocrf.org

Ovarian Cancer National Alliance
1627 K Street, N.W., 12th Floor
Washington, D.C. 20006
202-331-1332
web site: www.ovariancancer.org

National Ovarian Cancer Coalition
500 N.E. Spanish River Blvd., Suite 14
Boca Raton, FL 33431
888-OVARIAN
web site: www.ovarian.org

Gilda Radner Familial Ovarian Cancer Registry
Elm and Carlton Streets
Buffalo, NY 14263
800-682-7426
web site: www.ovariancancer.com

Society of Gynecologic Oncologists
401 No. Michigan Avenue
Chicago, IL 60611
800-444-4441 (Hotline)
web site: www.sgo.org

Prostate Problems and **Prostate Cancer** (see separate section, Page 270)

Web Site
Women's Cancer Network (WCN):
www.wcn.org
- Free medical info
- Doctor listings

Constipation, Diarrhea, Incontinence
It seems that, with age, we become more focused on the routines of our bodies—from regular sleep to regular bowel movements. That's perfectly normal, because, as our bodies age, we become more fragile and less likely to stay up all night (as in our youth) or not as likely to be so busy that we haven't time for "the pause that refreshes." We need the "refreshing" to feel stable and fit.

But this is another area in which different people have different habits. There is no absolute "normal" or "average" standard by which you must measure yourself. You measure yourself by your own routine, as long as there is one.

Constipation is not the world's most fascinating topic for conversation, but you can bet that it is a vital matter for us all. And, while some people have bowel movements (BMs) only two or three times a week, others are more regular at once a day. But there is no rule for everyone. That's why constipation is defined simply as "...having fewer bowel movements than usual." Sometimes, when BMs are not as often as is your habit, they take longer and are harder to do.

The questions to ask yourself, if you are concerned, are:
- Do you have fewer than 3 BMs a week?
- Do you have a hard time passing stools?
- Is there pain associated with having a BM?
- Is there any bleeding while having a BM?

Poor diet and dehydration are probably the biggest causes of constipation. But pro-biotics (as contrasted to antibiotics), such as fruits, vegetables, whole grains, and yogurt, are foods that aid good digestion (digestive facilitators). Conversely, eating lots of fats, dairy products, eggs, and sugars (deserts) can bring on constipation. People who live alone often don't cook for themselves; some eat processed or convenience foods, heated in a microwave, that are often low in fiber. And many people do not drink enough liquids, which add bulk to stools, making BMs easier. Lack of liquid intake (or dehydration) can be a major problem for older adults, particularly the frail elderly.

Other potential contributors to constipation are certain medications (read the labels) and the misuse of laxatives by people who think, incorrectly, that laxatives are a cure for constipation. There are even those who take laxatives every day, thinking that they will make them regular, when in fact the body adjusts to laxatives, which then become habit-forming. This can lead to diarrhea—simply trading one problem for another.

Most doctors counsel that, if you can, you should remain physically active, using your body and muscles. This allows for function, as contrasted to lack of exercise or too much bed-rest, which can cause constipation. While diarrhea is the opposite of constipation—and both can be brought under control—many older adults and elderly people worry more about incontinence, defined as "...unable to restrain a natural discharge." Incontinence is usually associated with one's bowels, but it can affect other bodily functions, such as urination.

Incontinence relates to the muscular function of the body, which naturally restrains the passing of bowels and urine until you are ready. For bowels, it is the sphincter muscle in the anus that performs that function. If that muscle weakens with age, you may be less able to control it; hence, there will be discharge when you don't want it. It has nothing to do with whether you are constipated, experiencing diarrhea, or having normal bowel movements. It has to do with muscle control and is referred to because it mostly affects the bowels.

There are protections against the effects of incontinence so that people can interact normally with each other without evidence of the problem. Most health care professionals are aware of these aids and can advise you regarding their use. Most importantly, you should not feel alone if you experience incontinence. It's not talked about a lot (understandably), but it is more common with age than reported. No one is a lesser or different person because of incontinence. It's simply a fact of life.

For More Information...

National Digestive Diseases Information Clearinghouse
Box NDDIC,
Bethesda, MD 20892
301-654-3810

Dental Care

Some people consider dental care secondary in their attention to health care. Perhaps that's because your teeth seem to be a more resilient part of your body. But those who act in this fashion do so at great risk.

Your mouth is the gateway for all the food you eat and the liquids you drink—and your teeth provide the initial stage of digestion, not to mention the first impression another person gets of your smile. If you consider your stomach integral to your body's absorption and use of food, your teeth are just as important. Most people understand this maxim if they experience a painful toothache, which can be more excruciating than a stomachache.

Most people are familiar with tooth decay, which causes cavities. But cavities are not just for children; they can be a factor as long as there are natural teeth in your mouth. For senior adults, the best way to protect against cavities is to have enough minerals in your diet and to avoid carbonated sodas. As far as your teeth are concerned, there is no redeeming value in colas!

Gum (periodontal) disease also can be a health factor among older adults. That's where the decay gets between your teeth and gums, often causing inflammation and bleeding. When gums are weak, the bone structure, which holds teeth in place, can be "lost." As is the case with all bone loss, tissue disintegrates. This could mean that teeth are loosened and, in the worst cases, may even fall out.

What's the best prevention? Brushing and flossing! Every dentist and dental hygienist preaches brushing and flossing regularly (try an electric toothbrush, if you can). Even lightly brush your tongue, they say, to remove food debris and make your mouth feel fresh. Flossing is important because it gets at the plaque your toothbrush cannot reach. But if you have bleeding gums, pain or irritation, see your dentist.

Other dental conditions to look for include dry mouth (xerostoma) and oral cancer. Dry mouth is more prevalent among older people and may make eating, drinking, and swallowing difficult. Basically, the salivary glands dry up, often due to prescription drugs used to combat other maladies. But you can combat dry mouth by drinking liquids and avoiding excesses of sugar, caffeine, tobacco, and alcohol.

Oral cancer is mostly an after-40 disease. As with most cancers, early detection means better treatment—before the spread of the cancer. Red or white patches on the gums or tongue, sores that don't heal, and difficulty chewing or swallowing are warning signs. The pathway to early detection, of course, is regular visits to your dentist. Don't wait for pain before you call the dentist, because that inhibits early detection, when oral cancer is curable. If you smoke cigarettes, use tobacco products, or drink excessive amounts of alcohol, you are at increased risk of developing oral cancer.

For More Information...

The National Institute of Dental Research (NIDR)
Building 31, Room 2C35
31 Center Drive, MSC 2290
Bethesda, MD 20892-2290
301-496-4261

National Oral Health Information Clearing House
1 NOHIC Way
Bethesda, MD 20892-3500
301-402-7364

American Dental Association
211 East Chicago Avenue
Chicago, IL 60611
800-621-8099

Older adults are more likely to wear dentures or partial dentures (false teeth). Those who do should keep dentures clean, just like natural teeth. Brushing all the surfaces with a denture-care product and removing dentures to let them soak in a cleansing liquid while you sleep are vital techniques.

Dentures, of course, may seem awkward when first worn, but most of the discomfort is a matter of adjusting. If eating, talking, or wearing dentures still seems difficult after a few weeks, consult your dentist.

If you are a candidate for dental implants (anchoring replacement teeth to your jawbone), be sure that your dentist is experienced, and discuss your condition and concerns with him or her thoroughly. The healing process for implants takes longer than dentures, so you will want to know what will happen and how you can assist your own healing.

Depression

In its 1994, 4th Edition of the *Diagnostic and Statistical Manual of Mental Disorders (DSM-IV)*, the American Psychiatric Association defines depression as lasting for at least two weeks, during which a patient experiences mood disturbances that last most of the day, along with at least four of the following symptoms:

- Depressed mood (feeling sad)
- Diminished interest in pleasure
- Significant weight loss
- Insomnia
- Psychomotor agitation or retardation
- Fatigue
- Feelings of worthlessness or guilt

- Difficulty with concentration
- Thoughts of death

It has been estimated (in a 1993 study entitled *Depression in Primary Care...Clinical Practice Guideline*, published by the U.S. Department of Health and Human Services) that depression is a factor in almost 25 percent of the general population (but only about half those are diagnosed or treated). Depression affects less than 10 percent of older adults in general; but among those in nursing homes, the figure rises to 25 percent.

Patients in the general population with chronic illness are at the highest risk for depression, but the elderly suffer chronic illnesses disproportionately. It makes sense, then, to be on the lookout for depression among those with chronic conditions, especially those in nursing homes.

Regular exercise, therapy, and mild antidepressants (given with special attention to avoiding adverse reactions to other prescribed drugs) are treatments for depression. Studies show that, after three episodes of depression among those on maintenance treatment, the rate of relapse is only 20 percent.

For More Information...

Depression and Related Affective Disorders Association (DRADA)
Meyer 3-181, 600 North Wolfe Street
Baltimore, MD 21287-7381
410-955-4647 (Baltimore, MD)
202-955-5800 (Washington DC)

Diabetes (Diabetes Mellitus)

In 1997, the American Board of Family Practice (one of the 26 recognized specialty boards for physicians) published its 6th Edition of the *Diabetes Mellitus Reference Guide*. Coupled with the 3rd Edition of the American Diabetes Association's *Therapy for Diabetes Mellitus and Related Disorders*, it offers the following sobering statistics on what we know simply as diabetes:

- In the general population, diabetes is the cause for 2.3 million hospital admissions (1997, the most recent complete data).
- This adds up to 14 million hospital days and 70 million nursing home days.
- The prevalence of diabetes is high in the general population—approximately 16 million cases, with more than half a million new cases each year (half of which go undiagnosed).
- Prevalence rises dramatically with age; more than 10 percent of persons over 65 have clinical diabetes. These 10 percent are at twice the risk for heart attacks and strokes as those without diabetes.

Treatments for diabetes, even for the elderly, are well within reach. The main treatment, of course, is glycemic control; that is, controlling the amount of sugar in the blood stream, primarily through a diet prescribed for the level of diabetic diagnosis. The more advanced the diabetes, the more restricted the diet. And, along with diet should go an effective exercise regimen.

Also, the 1998 United Kingdom Prospective Diabetes Study showed that controlling high blood pressure (hypertension) leads to significant reductions in deaths due to diabetes, strokes, and heart disease. Perhaps of greatest interest was the fact that control of hypertension in this study was as vital to these reductions as glycemic control. The study also demonstrated that lowering cholesterol levels is important.

For More Information...

American Diabetes Association
1701 North Beauregard Street
Alexandria, VA 22311
Diabetes Information and Action Line (DIAL):
800-DIABETES (800-342-2383)

Eye Care

Your eyes are your window to the world; they should never be taken for granted. Ask someone who is blind, and they will tell you how lucky you are to have your sight (even though they may have skills and insight that you would be lucky to have).

And, while there are many examples of people with excellent eyesight into their 80s and beyond, the fact is that growing older means that it may be more difficult to see without assistance. The most obvious example is the need to have glasses to adjust for near-or far-sightedness or for reading. Some people need bifocals for multiple adjustment. And, of course, eyeglasses come in all sizes, shapes, and fashions. They're big business.

We joke about reaching the age when we need glasses, but the truth for most of us is that we do reach an age when, without glasses, we wouldn't function as well. That's the easy part. The more difficult matters relating to eye care for older adults are cataracts, complications of diabetes, and glaucoma.

Cataracts grow painlessly and gradually over one or both eyes and are the cause of cloudiness or blurred vision that impairs reading ability and driving. Cataracts can be removed surgically, and a new lens (intraocular) can be installed. The success rate for this surgery is one of the highest.

Recommendations

- Get an eye checkup every one-two years; most eye conditions can be treated when they are found early.
- Take extra care if you have a family history of eye disease; have an eye exam once a year.

A side effect of diabetes is a buildup of fluid in the retina of the eye or the growth of blood cells in the eye that can rupture and form scar tissue. Again, however, for those with diabetes, these issues can be addressed by changing medications and diet.

Glaucoma, a group of eye diseases that manifest themselves in increased pressure in the fluid of the eye, can be serious. Glaucoma can even lead to blindness, if left untreated. If you have an eye examination every two years, as most experts recommend, you can catch glaucoma in its early stages and treat it with drugs or surgery, if needed.

There is a list of other complaints relating to the eye. Each have varying degrees of seriousness, but the advice common to all of them is to see an eye doctor. All of these complaints are treatable, but treatment is more difficult when the condition is advanced:

- Floaters—tiny spots that float in your field of vision,
- Dry Eyes—the tear glands don't create enough liquid,
- Tearing—too many tears, often caused by wind or changes in temperatures,
- Retinal Disorders—afflictions to the retina, which is a thin lining in the back of the eye (retinal disorders are the leading cause of blindness),
- Macular Degeneration—usually age-related deterioration of the millions of cells in the center of the eye that are sensitive to light, thus impairing clarity of vision,
- Conjunctivitis—when the lining of the eyelid becomes inflamed, causing itching, burning, or tearing, or the feeling that there is something in your eye,
- Corneal Diseases—damage to the cornea, the curved "window" in front of the eye that helps to focus light as it enters; if the damage results in loss of sight, cornea transplants can be done surgically, with a high success rate,
- Eyelid Problems—including drooping eyelids, can be corrected by surgery or medications, and
- Temporal Arteritis—inflammation of the arteries in the temple of the forehead, which causes headaches and some pain; it can also cause sud-

den loss of vision, which can be treated with pre-scription drugs (the earlier, the better).

And, it stands to reason, if you experience any dimming or loss of eyesight, eye pain, leaking fluids from your eye, double vision, or swelling of your eye or eyelid, see an eye doctor right away.

For More Information...

The National Eye Institute
2020 Vision Place
Bethesda, MD 20892-3655
301-496-5248

The American Optometric Association
243 North Lindbergh Boulevard
St. Louis, MO 63141
314-991-4100

The American Foundation for the Blind
11 Penn Plaza, Suite 300
New York, NY 10001
800-334-5497

The Lighthouse National Center for Vision and Aging
11 East 59th Street
New York, NY 10022
212-821-9705

The National Association for the Visually Handicapped
22 West 21st Street
New York, NY 10010
212-889-3141

The National Eye Care Project of the American Academy of Ophthalmology (AAO)
P.O. Box 6988
San Francisco, CA 94120-6988
800-222-EYES

The National Library Service for the Blind and Physically Handicapped
1291 Taylor Street, N.W.
Washington, D.C. 20542
800-424-8567

The National Society to Prevent Blindness
500 East Remington Road
Schaumburg, IL 60173-5611
800-331-2020

The Vision Foundation
818 Mr. Auburn Street
Watertown, MA 02172
617-926-4232

The National Institute on Aging
P.O. Box 8057
Gaithersburg, MD 20898-8057
800-222-2225

Flu: Getting Your Shots

Flu is short for *influenza*, a virus you don't want to catch, especially if you are older. It can be life threatening in older adults who have chronic diseases (heart disease, emphysema, asthma, bronchitis, kidney disease, or diabetes). The flu attacks the nose, throat, and lungs and impairs your ability to fight infections. It can lead to pneumonia.

But you can prevent the flu! According to the Administration on Aging's web site (www.aoa.dhhs.gov/aoa/pages/agepages/flu.html), "...people over 50 *need* to get a flu shot every year." Notice it says "need," not "should" or "may." It's simple: Get the shot—Prevent the flu! Don't get the shot—You risk misery for days at the least! Most communities have flu shot clinics every year in the fall, and the cost of the shot is approximately $5.

There are many strains of flu—some are imported through normal contact between people from areas all over the world. We are not alone in dealing with the flu. But in the U.S., each year the Centers for Disease Control (CDC) identifies the origins of the flu, predicts the type of flu that will invade that season, and organizes production of supplies of vaccines to combat the most prevalent flu predicted.

Don't confuse the flu with the common cold. While symptoms vary, a cold doesn't usually cause fever; the flu does. Colds mean stuffy noses; that's rare with the flu. Colds go away sooner; the flu, with its fever, chills (sometimes shaking chills), aching muscles, headaches, coughing, and watery eyes, hangs around longer. Who needs it? Who wants it?

But if you get the flu, the treatment is the adage ascribed to physicians: "Take an aspirin and call me in the morning." Well, not quite literally, particularly if a fever persists. Yes, take aspirin, but also drink plenty of liquids and get bed rest, even for a day or two after the fever is gone. For high-risk people, there are prescription drugs your doctor can prescribe to alleviate serious symptoms.

In its bulletin, "Shots for Safety," the National Institute on Aging recommends a one-time pneumonia prevention shot for people over 65, a booster shot for tetanus and diphtheria every ten years, and vaccinations against measles, mumps, rubella, and hepatitis B, particularly if you work with young people. These shots should be a part of your regular health care regimen, and you should keep a record of them and carry that record in your wallet or purse.

For a free copy of a booklet entitled *Immunization of Adults: A Call To Action*, contact: The Centers for Disease Control and Prevention, 1600 Clifton Road, Atlanta, GA 30333, 404-639-8225. For a free copy of the booklet *Flu*, contact the National Institute of Allergy and Infectious Diseases, 9000 Rockville Pike, Bethesda, MD 20892, 301-496-5717. Or for more information, contact The National Institute on Aging Information Center, P.O. Box 8057, Gaithersburg, MD 20898-8057, 800-222-2225.

Foot Care

The older you get, the more important your feet seem to be to you. Soothing your aching feet might have been an expression you used after a long day of standing at a counter or working as a waitress, but, as you age, your feet seem to ache just from walking, and they seem to need soothing more. That's normal and natural.

For the most part, when it comes to foot care, you are your own best doctor. But if your feet have been abused, you will want to consult a podiatrist (foot doctor) or your primary care physician for treatment. Plain old tired, aching feet can have serious problems if you have worn badly designed or poorly fitting shoes for years or you have poor circulation in your feet. Also, if your toenails have not been trimmed often enough or properly, your feet will suffer.

The antidotes for these maladies are comfortable, well-fitting shoes (perhaps the most important) and exercise, raising your feet up, standing, walking, gentle massage, and warm foot baths to improve circulation. And, of course, trim your toenails, lest they impair the comfort of your shoes.

Other common foot problems are:

- Athlete's Foot—a fungal, bacterial condition, treated by fungicidal powder or spray after cleaning,
- Dry skin—Itching and a burning sensation, treated by mild soap and body lotion,
- Corns and calluses—caused by friction, are best treated by a podiatrist or physician (over-the-counter drugs containing acid destroy the tissue but not the cause),
- Warts—caused by viruses, painful if untreated, should be removed only by a podiatrist or physician by applications of medicines, burning or freezing the wart off, or surgical removal,
- Bunions—develop when big toe joints are out of

line; they are tender and painful and are treated by a wider shoe fit, protective pads, injecting drugs, or, in some cases, surgery,

- Ingrown toenails—happen when toenails are not trimmed correctly and the toenail breaks the skin of the toe; your podiatrist or physician can remove the offending part of the toenail, allowing the wound to heal,

- Hammertoe—caused by shortening of the tendons that control toe movement, and is treated by more loosely fitting shoes and socks or stockings or, in advanced cases, surgery, and

- Spurs—deposits of calcium on the bones of your feet; they are sometimes quite painful and are treated by proper foot support such as heel pads and heel cups.

For More Information...

The American Podiatric Medical Association
9312 Old Georgetown Road
Bethesda, MD 20814

The American Orthopedic Foot and Ankle Society
2517 Eastlake Avenue E
Seattle, WA 98102
206-223-1120

National Institute on Aging (NIH)
Building 31, Room 5C27
31 Center Drive, MSC2292
Bethesda, MD 20892
301-496-1752

Wearing comfortable shoes is probably the best favor you can do for yourself and your feet. The width of your feet will increase with age, so it's important, when buying shoes, to measure your feet carefully. Shop for soles that will enhance solid footing and not be slippery. Thick soles will cushion your feet on hard surfaces. Low-heeled shoes are more comfortable and safer than high-heeled shoes. High heels may be fashionable, but they are unnatural for your feet. If you wear high heels, do so infrequently and for short periods.

Hearing and Hearing Loss

Most hearing problems are minor, but it's easy to get a little irritated when you miss something or don't quite hear a sentence correctly. If you don't hear the doorbell, you might miss a package you were expecting. Hearing loss can worsen as we get older, but that's almost an expected part of life.

Almost a third of people over 65 have some hearing problems, and half of those over 85 do. Some of these problems can be quite serious, causing the impaired person to withdraw from contact with others in order to avoid feeling embarrassed because communication is difficult. When this happens, it may seem that older adults are confused, forgetful, or unresponsive; but the truth is, they just don't hear well.

But hearing loss can be corrected. A physician can prescribe special training, hearing aids, medicines, or even surgery. You don't have to live with hearing loss, if you act. The National Institute on Aging suggests the following warning signs:

- Words are hard to understand.

- Another person's speech sounds slurred or mumbled, especially when there is background noise.
- Certain sounds are overly annoying or seem loud.
- A hissing or ringing in the background is heard.
- TV shows, concerts, and parties are less enjoyable because you cannot hear much.

If these signs appear, see your physician, who may suggest that you be measured by an audiologist, a health professional who can identify hearing loss, or an otolaryngologist, a doctor who specializes in ears, nose, and throat. These professionals can often determine the cause of hearing loss: extended exposure to loud noises, head injuries, tumors, reaction to certain medicines, viral or bacterial infections, heart conditions or stroke, or changes in the ear that are a result of aging.

The most common types of hearing loss are presbycusis, a loss of hearing linked to the inner ear, and tinnitus, a ringing, roaring, or other sound inside the ears. Tinnitus can be caused by wax buildup, an ear infection, reaction to certain medicines, a nerve disorder, a benign tumor in the inner ear, or a host of other reasons. Often the reason for the ringing cannot be found, and it often goes away by itself.

If you have trouble hearing, say so to others, so they can talk more clearly and use facial expressions and gestures. And, above all, be patient with your malady. Stay involved and included, especially if your hearing loss is the matter under discussion. Don't allow yourself to feel isolated. Ask if your words are being understood.

And, of course, you can get a small device that fits in your ear and magnifies sound—a hearing aid. Many hearing aids today are attractive and function much better than earlier models. Before you purchase a hearing aid, you must obtain a written evaluation of your hearing or sign a waiver saying you don't want the evaluation.

When you buy a hearing aid, you must have full information on the fitting of the aid, directions for its use, and repairs during the warranty period. An evaluation is advised because the type of hearing aid prescribed depends on the diagnosis (hairs in ears, wax buildup, nerve degeneration, hardening of the eardrum, or ossification of the ear canal).

For More Information...

The American Academy of Otolaryncology, Head, and Neck Surgery
One Prince Street
Alexandria, VA 22314
703-836-4444 or 703-519-1585 (TTY)

The American Speech-Language-Hearing Association
10801 Rockville Pike, Dept. AP
Rockville, MD 20852
Hotline: 800-638-8255 (Voice/TTY)

Heart Disease
If the proportion of the elderly is supposed to increase by 50 percent in the next 30 years, then it is vital to apply the brakes to heart disease (ischemic heart dis-

ease or coronary artery disease)—a condition that disproportionately affects the older population. The American Heart Association says, in its *1998 Heart and Stroke Statistical Update*, that heart disease is the number one cause of death among elderly patients.

Heart failure and heart disease are closely related and share statistics from the American Heart Association and the National Center for Health Statistics. Consider: 16 percent of Americans 65 and older have heart disease. There are 1.5 million cases of myocardial infarction (heart attack) and angina pectoris (unstable angina) each year; 60 percent of those involve persons over 65.

But heart disease does not have to lead to heart failure, even into later years (75-80). In several clinical trials, cholesterol-lowering drugs have been proven to benefit patients with coronary artery disease. So has plain old aspirin, even among hospitalized patients, as well as those living independently. For acute patients, beta blocker and thrombolytic therapies can measurably improve the mortaility rate.

Yet, it appears from other studies that the use of these "therapies" is not common, even though the benefits have been documented and even advertised. For example, it is now well-known that taking an 81 mg aspirin a day (all major stores sell aspirin in an 81 mg dose) will help stem the onset of heart disease, but how many people do so? (NOTE: Check with your doctor. Aspirin can cause internal bleeding in the case of some diagnosed conditions.)

> Take an 81 mg aspirin a day (all other health con-
> ditions being equal) and consult your doctor
> about other therapies if you are diagnosed with
> heart disease, particularly the benefit of lower-
> ing cholesterol. Stick to a low fat diet and exer-
> cise!

Heart Failure

It is standard procedure for physicians to prescribe a heavy dose of quality-of-life changes when a patient is diagnosed with heart failure (the inability of the heart to pump enough blood to adequately supply body tissues). None of these prescriptions should be a surprise; it's just that heart failure can be the "wake-up call" that shouldn't have been necessary, but apparently is. The prescription?

- Monitoring Weight Daily; A Low Fat Diet
- Strict Medication Management
- Restriction on Salt Intake; Increase Vitamin B6
- Exercise Training (An Exercise Regime)
- NO SMOKING!
- Counseling for Patient and Family

Physicians will also prescribe medications that can reduce the onset of new/repeat heart failure and reduce the number of deaths from heart failure. (According to several articles in the *New England Journal of Medicine* from 1992 to 1996, this includes ACE inhibitor therapy and beta blocker therapy for patients with moderate to severe dysfunction of the left ventricular system.)

In addition, there is treatment for lowering blood pressure (hypertension) and cholesterol (lipid lowering therapy) that can reduce the risk of developing heart failure among the elderly.

Physicians are aggressive about treating heart failure. In the general population, there are 4.6 million heart failure patients (*1999 Heart and Stroke Statistical Update*, American Heart Association). The estimated direct annual cost of hospitalization and treatment is $19.6 billion! And the prevalence of heart failure increases with age. Heart failure affects 5 percent of those aged 60 to 69, and 10 percent of those aged 70 and older). The overall fatality rate from heart failure is 20 percent in the first year after diagnosis and 50 percent within five years. The older the patient, the greater the mortality rate after diagnosis, especially those patients who are hospitalized.

For More Information...

American Heart Association
7272 Greenville Avenue
Dallas, TX 75231
Heart and Stroke Info Line: 800-AHA-USA1

Hormone Replacement Therapy (Osteoporosis and Menopause)

Hormone Replacement Therapy (HRT) is a subject on which volumes have been written and about which we still have much to learn. This much we do know: the body's natural hormonal balance changes as we age, and there are certain times in life, especially for women, when such changes are noticeable, such as during menopause.

Menopause is the stage in a woman's life when menstruation stops as a result of her body making less of the female hormones, estrogen and progesterone. While this is natural for *all* women, *some* women experience moderate to severe discomfort, including hot flashes (sudden flushes of warmth, even sweating), disruption of sleeping habits, vaginal dryness resulting in uncomfortable (or even painful) sex, changes in sexual desire, headaches, and lower tolerance of stress.

Estrogen loss can mean bone loss and even osteoporosis. The rise in osteoporosis, which now affects 24 million people in the United States, may account for

---

The Estrogen Dilemma

If you are a woman nearing menopause, you should take estrogen-progestin. But for how long? That depends on the severity of your symptoms, your lifestyle, and your family health history.

Short-term Benefits
- Cools hot flashes
- Combats insomnia
- Counters vaginal dryness
- Smooths out mood swings

Long-term Benefits
- Retards osteoporosis
- Reduces the risk of heart disease
- Neutralizes the risk of uterine cancer
- May reduce the risk of Alzheimer's disease and colon cancer

Long-term Risks
- Increases the risk of breast cancer
- Promotes the formation of gallstones and blood clots

–Time, Vol 155, No 5, February 7, 2000

higher risk of heart disease and stroke, the leading causes of death among women over 50.

For women weathering the effects of menopause, physicians often prescribe "hormone replacement" to alter the "mix" of natural estrogen and progesterone. Habitually, doctors prescribe estrogen alone for those women who have had a hysterectomy, and estrogen combined with progestin to relieve adverse symptoms of menopause or prevent bone loss.

Note, however, that progestin is a chemical synthetic developed to mimic the body's natural progesterone. The two are not "bio-identical." In fact, one recent study suggests that progestin, combined with estrogen, may increase the risk of cancer. The study is debatable, but there is little debate that progesterone is natural and poses no risks.

In some cases, doctors prescribe a mix of estrogen for a number of days, add progestin for another set of days, and then stop for a specific time in an attempt to mimic a regular menstrual cycle. But most prescriptions call for a constant dosage of a mix that stops any monthly bleeding.

For More Information...

Hormone Replacement Therapy
PreventingOsteoporosis
The Menopause Years
The American College Of Obstetricians and Gynocologists (ACOG)
409 12th Street, S.W.
Washington, DC 20024-2188

Continued

Hormone Replacement Therapy: Facts to Help You Decide
AARP Women's Initiative
601 E Street, N.W.
Washington, DC 20049
800-424-3410

As beneficial as hormone replacement therapy is, warnings against taking HRT are pronounced if you have high blood pressure, diabetes, liver disease, blood clots, seizures, migraine headaches, gall bladder disease, or a history of cancer.

Risks include cancer of the uterus (endometrial cancer) for women who take estrogen alone, although today physicians usually prescribe "opposition" (meaning an offset) to estrogen by combining it with progestin.

Another risk in taking HRT, depending on the therapy chosen, is increased risk of breast cancer.

A recent report in the *Journal of the American Medical Association* links estrogen therapy (alone), and estrogen combined with progestin, with significantly higher incidents of breast cancer (20 percent and 40 percent, respectively).

Organiztions to Contact

**The National Resource Center On
Osteoporosis and Related Bone Diseases**
800-624-BONE

The North American Menopause Society
P.O. Box 94527
Cleveland, OH 44101
440-442-7550

The National Women's Health Network
514 10th Street, N.W.
Washington, DC 20004
202-347-1140

The Older Women's League
666 11th Street, N.W., #700
Washington, DC 20001
202-783-6686

The National Cancer Institute
Building 31, Room 10A03
31 Center Drive, MSC2580
Bethesda, MD 20892
800-4-CANCER or 301-435-3848

The National Heart, Lung and Blood Institute
301-251-1222

In her February, 2000, article on the results of this study, *Time* reporter J. Madeleine Nash wrote, "'Poor women!' sighs University of Michigan cardiologist Dr.

Lori Mosca. 'Every time a new study comes out, they have to revisit the decision they've made.' There are 8.6 million women in the nation now taking the estrogen-progestin combination."

Side effects can include headaches, nausea, vaginal discharge, fluid retention, swollen breasts, weight gain, and slowing of digestion.

On the other hand, studies have repeatedly demonstrated that taking estrogen alone lowers the risk of heart disease or stroke in women over 50, when they are otherwise most at risk. The estrogen and progestin combination can also reduce the risk of heart disease.

If you take HRT, the American College of Obstetricians and Gynecologists says that you should get a medical checkup once a year.

At that time, you should get a pelvic and breast examination and have a mammogram.

And remember, in HRT: One size does NOT fit all. Simple blood tests can be used to measure the individual "mix" of hormones in your own body so that an HRT regime that fits you personally can be prescribed—a regime that now comes in the form of patches and creams as well as shots and pills.

And remember, too: You may choose to decline HRT. If so, there are good health habits you can adopt to deal with the adverse symptoms of menopause. There are drugs that can reduce hot flashes, and you can simply lower the room temperature at night to help you sleep.

To help build the strength of your bones, make sure you get 1,000 mg of calcium each day (after menopause, 1,500 mg) by drinking low-fat milk and by eating dairy foods and yogurt. In addition, your diet should include enough minerals, whole grains, etc. to help rebuild bone strength. This includes magnesium—to be taken with calcium—silicon, and boron. These can be taken as a supplement, but it is better to make them a part of your regular diet.

By doing regular weight-bearing exercise (when your muscles work against gravity), you can strengthen your muscles which, in turn, can relieve the pressure of weight on your bones and help in preventing osteoporosis. This type of exercise can be as simple as walking or running, and it can build strength right on the bone itself through the blood stream, adding minerals to both bone and cartilage.

And there are other options, aside from HRT, for preventing heart disease and bone loss. There's a new drug to treat osteoporosis in women past menopause that you can ask your doctor about. In fact, it would be wise to discuss with your doctor all relevant risks and benefits of HRT, both short-term and long-term.

But, as Nash points out, there are trade-offs: "A woman whose family history places her at risk for breast cancer might decide to avoid hormone therapy even for the short term…while a woman at high risk for osteoporosis or heart disease would probably be more willing to take her chances."

Pain Management (Chronic Pain)

Pain management, which generally applies to chronic pain, is a subject that has come into its own over the past ten years. Physicians today are less inhibited about prescribing drugs to manage long-term pain. At some level, 25-40 percent of those over 65 experience pain on a daily basis. For those over 65 who are in nursing homes, the rate is 70-80 percent.

Many people do not report their pain. But the severe consequences of ignoring chronic pain can lead to depression, social isolation, sleep deprivation, and decreased mobility—all of which add to increased need for health care treatment and added costs, of course.

For many years, doctors were afraid to prescribe pain-killing drugs on a regular basis, because the pattern of prescriptions might raise suspicions that they were feeding a patient's addiction.

In California, this obvious conflict grew to the point where the State Medical Board,

> ### *Chronic or Acute Pain*
>
> **Chronic pain** is that which is long lasting and recurring as a result of an illness, condition, or disease.
>
> **Acute pain** is sharp, severe, and very serious; a result of an injury or internal cramp or stabbing sensation.

charged with licensure and discipline of physicians, launched studies leading to a summit conference of experts, which, in turn, led to the adoption and publication of "pain management guidelines." The guidelines describe a step-by-step patient process, which, if followed and documented by prescribing physicians, renders them free from suspicion or doubt and allows them to perform as "healers" to their patients in need of treatment.

In addition, those same physicians continue to recommend non-drug therapy such as stress reduction and relaxation, which have always been factors in reducing chronic pain. Reduction of stress actually changes the pain-causing chemicals in the body. And, almost anything we can do to take our minds off our pain will provide a level of relaxation that, in the long run, can be a real benefit.

Guidelines on Prescribing

**Medical Board of California,
Adopted Unanimously, July 29, 1994**

"No physician and surgeon shall be subject to disciplinary action by the board for prescribing or administering controlled substances in the course of treatment of a person for intractable pain."

— Business and Professions Code, Section 2241.5
Statutes of the State of California

1. A medical history and physical examination of the patient must be accomplished, including an assessment of pain, physical and psychological function, substance abuse history, an assessment of underlying or coexisting diseases or conditions and should include presence of a recognized medical indication for the use of a controlled substance.

2. There should be a treatment plan, which should state objectives by which treatment can be evaluated ... and the physician should tailor drug therapy to the individual medical needs of each patient.

Continued

3. The physician should discuss the risks and benefits of the use of controlled substances with the patient or guardian.

4. The physician should periodically review the course of opioid treatment and any new information about the etiology of the pain....If the patient has not improved, the physician should assess the appropriateness of continued opioid treatment or trial of other modalities.

5. The physician should be willing to refer the patient for additional evaluation and treatment in order to achieve treatment objectives...especially patients with a history of substance abuse...

6. The physician should keep accurate and complete records according to items 1-5, above.

7. The physician must be properly licensed to practice medicine and to prescribe controlled substances in accordance with federal and state laws and regulations.

Getting to the level of controlling pain with narcotic drug prescriptions is not taken lightly by physicians. While many medicines can control pain, they also have side effects, some of which can be serious. This is the time, therefore, to "team" with your doctor and your pharmacist. Be straightforward with them, describe your pain as precisely as you can, ask questions about side effects, and listen carefully to instructions, particularly if you are taking medicines for other conditions.

A recent information sheet (updated in March, 2000), published by the American Academy of Family Practice, divides pain control drugs into three main categories: acetaminophens, anti-inflammatory drugs, and narcotics.

The most common over-the-counter medicine taken to control pain is acetaminophen (Tylenol, Panadol, etc.), too much of which can cause damage to your liver. When you buy an acetaminophen, remember that some other over-the-counter drugs you may be taking for other reasons may also contain acetaminophen (read the label or ask your pharmacist); the combinations may be harmful.

Anti-inflammatory drugs to control the pain of swelling (aspirin and ibuprofen, such as Advil, Motrin, Nuprin, etc., and naproxen, such as Naprosyn, Aleve, etc.) should be taken with food or milk because the most common side effects impact the stomach. The effect of anti-inflammatory drugs taken over time is not only to reduce the pain, but also to reduce swelling.

When needed, narcotic drugs can be prescribed, usually starting with low doses and increasing doses as necessary. It is vital that you closely follow your doctor's instructions when taking these drugs. They are an important part of your therapy to control pain, but they can become physically or psychologically addicting. Side effects can include an inability to concentrate or think clearly. Usually your doctor will tell you not to drive a car when you're taking narcotic drugs.

There is no need to fear addiction as a consequence of taking narcotic drugs if you are careful and monitor yourself in accordance with physician instructions.

There are two kinds of addiction: physical and psychological. Physical dependence develops when your body gets used to the routine ingestion of a drug and needs the drug in order to function. Psychological addiction is evident when you have a strong desire to use the drug, whether or not your body needs it.

If you have a physical dependence alone, then when your pain diminishes, your doctor can help you slowly reduce your intake until the pain is gone (your body no longer needs the drug). Psychological addiction can be dangerous, and it probably won't ease your pain. Your doctor may prescribe a different drug, lower the dose, or stop the prescription altogether. Counseling also may be advised.

A common side effect of using narcotic drugs is constipation. Left unattended, this condition can be a serious consequence. Yet, it is relatively easy to deal with by drinking six to eight glasses of water a day and eating six to eight servings of fruit and vegetables. If problems persist, check with your doctor. A laxative may be in order, but ask first.

There are other drugs that are used for other conditions that may also help in controlling pain. One example is a seizure medication (carbamazepine, aka Tegretol). Another is an antidepressant (amitripyline, aka Elavil or Endep). Be advised, however, that these medicines can take weeks to reach the stage at which they help control pain. Your doctor will advise you.

Controlling chronic or intractable pain has never been a simple matter for either the patient or the doctor. Today there are better tools to help the process, such as a "standard pain scale" used in evaluating results in trying to control pain in cancer patients. And it is clear in study after study that patients who are educated about their pain are far better at taking their medications and, as a result, show significant decreases in pain intensity, anxiety, and fear of addiction.

For more information, visit the American Academy of Family Practice's general web site: www.aafp.org/healthinfo. The AAFP also has a web site specific to inquiries about pain management: www.aafp.org/patientinfo/helppain.html

Pressure Ulcers

Pressure ulcers are commonly known as bed sores and are most often associated with stays in nursing homes as a result of long duration of bed rest. Indeed, The National Pressure Ulcer Advisory Panel, in its *Prevention Monograph* (www.npuap.org/prevmon.htm), says that 23 percent of all patients in nursing homes have pressure ulcers at any one time, but so do 11 percent of those in acute care hospitals.

In a 1993 article in the *American Family Physician*, entitled "Pressure Ulcers in Nursing Home Patients," authors G.D. Spoelhof and K. Ide point out that 11 percent of nursing home residents had pressure ulcers at the time of admission, 13 percent developed them within one year, and 22 percent developed them within two years.

Pressure ulcers cause discomfort and pain and can result in disfigurement, if they are not addressed. They can make daily living much more difficult for elderly patients, and they can predispose patients to osteomyletis and septicemia. If patients are hospitalized with broken bones or a fractured hip, it is even harder to prevent pressure ulcers. The risks are immobility or impaired mobility, incontinence, poor nutrition, and diminished mental awareness.

Significantly, the National Pressure Ulcer Advisory Panel, in February, 1999, published a paper by C. Lyder entitled "The Pressure Ulcer Challenge: Balancing Cost and Quality." Reference is made to this paper in a fact sheet entitled "New Facts About Pressure Ulcers in Older Adults," a joint publication by Pfizer U.S. Pharmaceuticals and The RAND Corporation. The author refers to the routine use of well-established risk assessment scales to predict probable pressure ulcer incidents. Lyder states that nursing homes that used the scales "...experienced less than half the pressure ulcer incidence than those that did not." The experience was similar in hospitals. One wonders why all nursing homes and hospitals do not use the risk assessment scales!

Routinely, patients are helped by frequent repositioning, cleansing of wounds, and the application of topical dressings with a moist healing environment and ensuring adequate nutrition.

Prostate Problems and Prostate Cancer

Prostate problems occur most frequently in men over 50, but infections of the prostate can occur at any age. Prostate cancer is most common among men over 65 (80 percent). Early detection, which is difficult because of the prostate's location in the body, is key to effective treatment.

The prostate is a small organ (about the size of a walnut) located below the bladder and surrounding the urethra. Its function is to control the flow of urine and to make fluid that becomes part of semen, which contains sperm. That's why men often worry about sexual dysfunction when they have prostate problems, but most treatment can be rendered without impairing sexual activity.

There are two major prostate problems that can develop. One is acute prostatitis, a bacterial infection, which can cause fever, chills, and pain in the lower back and between the legs. Prostatitis can be treated with antibiotics, but it can become chronic, albeit with reduced pain and discomfort. In some instances, chronic prostatitis goes away by itself.

The other problem is benign prostatic hypertrophy (BPH). More than half of all men over 60 have BPH; and 90 percent of men over 70 have it. BPH is the enlargement of the prostate, which can be detected by a rectal examination. The chief symptom is difficulty in urinating (in rare cases, a patient may be unable to urinate), yet there may be the urge to urinate often. In such cases, a doctor (often a urologist) will examine a patient with a cytoscope, which is inserted into the penis to "see" the urethra, prostate, and bladder.

In the beginning, doctors and patients wait to see if the problem of BPH gets worse. In the meantime, a physician can prescribe drugs that help relax muscles and relieve symptoms, even shrink the prostate. Sometimes surgery, increasingly done with a surgical instrument inserted through the penis, is indicated. The surgeon removes part of the prostate to reduce the enlargement. Patients have choices about surgical procedures. To help, there is a booklet published by The Agency for Health Care Policy and Research, which is free. Call 800-358-9295.

Of all prostate cases, 80 percent occur in men over 65. The probability is that one man in ten will have prostate cancer by the time he reaches age 85. Diagnosed cases are on the rise, but that is not because there is an increased incidence; it is because of the aging of our population and earlier screening of patients. In a book sponsored by the American Cancer Society, *Prostate Cancer: What Every Man—And His Family—Needs to Know* (Villard Press, New York, 1996), three physician-authors (David G. Bostwick, Gregory T. MacLennan, and Thayne R. Larson) report that the incidence of prostate cancer in men is 33 percent greater than breast cancer in women.

But prostate cancer is not life threatening if it is detected early and has not spread beyond the prostate. It is difficult to detect, however, because of the location of the prostate deep inside the pelvis and surrounded by other organs. Yet diagnosis can be a simple matter of a rectal exam. When the physician inserts a finger into the rectum, he or she can feel the prostate. If a physician feels that the prostate is hard or unusually lumpy, that will lead to additional diagnostic steps—a blood test (prostate specific antigen [PSA]) or a biopsy (a simple surgical procedure) to test an actual tiny piece of the prostate.

According to authors Bostwick, McLennan, and Larson, the warning signs of prostate cancer are:

Urinary:
- Urgent need to urinate
- Frequent need to urinate
- Urination at night
- Urination is painful
- Urine leaks out without control

Obstructive:
- Difficulty getting urine started
- Weak or interrupted urinary stream
- Feeling that the bladder is full, even after urination

Others:
- Pain in the lower back or pelvic area
- Loss of appetite
- Unexplained weight loss

Taken in some combination, these warning signs should lead you to your doctor, who can conduct tests that can lead to diagnosis and treatment. Treatment may vary, depending on other medical conditions, your age, and your overall health. But most often, the treatment is surgical:

- Usually removing the entire prostate and surrounding tissues, but preserving sexual function (some men experience incontinence [can't control the need to urinate] after surgery, but that usually clears up in most patients in a few weeks).
- A transurethral resection, which cuts out the cancer without removing the entire prostate.
- Radiation using high-energy rays to kill the cancer cells and shrink tumors (here there is a risk of impotence, however).
- Hormone therapy, which can retard or stop the growth of cancer cells; hence, preventing the spread of the cancer.

For More Information...

The Agency for Health Care Policy and Research Publications Clearinghouse
P.O. Box 8547
Silver Spring, MD 20927
800-358-9295

The Cancer Information Center
National Cancer Institute
Building 31, Room 10A24
Bethesda, MD 20892
800-4CANCER

The National Kidney and Urologic Diseases Information Clearing House
Box NKUDIC
Bethesda, MD 20892
301-468-6345

Sexuality

Sexuality is probably one of the matters most older people worry about as they age, yet the worry causes more stress than the reality. Sexuality is ageless. The older you get, the more slowing of response there may be, but that is normal! But most people enjoy regular sex, if they want to, into advanced years without strain or thinking they have to "perform." Moreover, sexuality is much more than the act of intercourse. It's an act of giving, not taking. Touching and being touched can be a healing experience. Holding your partner can trigger a release of stored emotions, "letting go" of the day and relaxing into a restful sleep at night.

In fact, "performance"—seemingly so important in our youth—is not the issue at all (it never really has been). It's all about genuine attraction and being intimate. Being "loving," in a word—for "loving" and "being loved" is vital to us all. It effects everything about us, because it's a central part of the entirety of who we are. Just imagine what life would be like without love—everything from the simplest expression of regard or respect, to deep and abiding commitment that is the focus of your life.

Sexual expression is sweet and beautiful, tender and meaningful. It won't mirror the sexuality of our youth. In fact, it can be an emotional fullness never yet experienced. Sexuality, albeit different, can open up whole new worlds as you age. The difference can mean a shared spiritual focus with your partner that stimulates and energizes you both. Imagination and memory may broaden with age providing new depth to experience.

At the same time, there are clinical aspects to sexuality when you are aging that you should know about. And making provision or allowances will result in a more satisfying relationship.

There are physical changes that come with age. Women may notice a decrease in vaginal lubrication; there are over-the-counter lubricants for that. Men may notice what is called "erectile dysfunction," but there are ways of discovering the causative factors which can be treated. In addition, there are prescription drugs (Viagra, for example), that are widely used by hundreds of thousands of men with success.

For women, a hysterectomy can seem debilitating to sexual activity, but that may be more a matter of the mind. If that's the case, counseling can help. Otherwise, sexual function usually returns to normal after a reasonable post-surgery wait.

Local chapters of the American Cancer Society can help women who feel sexually impaired after a mastectomy. A mastectomy does not eliminate a woman's physical desire for sex. But some women experience feelings of being less than complete because of what they see as a disfigurement. Others feel inadequate, thinking they are less desirable; or they believe their partners see them as unattractive. In these cases, it helps to talk to other women who have experienced the same concerns and can share their feelings.

For men undergoing removal of their prostate (prostatectomy), the surgery rarely causes impotence. In radical cases, surgery can be performed so that the nerves that affect sexual activity are not touched. This is something that should be discussed with the surgeon and can be handled, in most cases, with relative ease.

There are other issues about which a straightforward approach is the best policy:

- Smoking and alcohol abuse reduce potency in men and delay orgasm in women.
- Some prescription drugs can reduce ejaculation in men and sexual desire in women. (Check with your physician or pharmacist.)
- Masturbation, which keeps sexual activity going, is helpful for people whose partners are ill or away and for unmarried, widowed, or divorced people.
- Having *safe* sex, with HIV and AIDS in mind, is essential at any age. If you are going to have sex

with a partner you do not know well and who may have other sexual partners, you *must* use a condom.

Worry about impotence and sexual function may very well cause the stress that can lead to impotence, even if there are no apparent physical reasons. Our societal emphasis on youth and beauty is not reality, but it can lead many people to draw comparisons to themselves, inhibit them from being outgoing or to try new experiences, and may even cause depression and lowering of self-esteem. How unnecessary!

Instead, take your time to appreciate another and yourself—together. Form a relationship that is built on an abiding interest in each other, that causes you naturally (with respect) to reach out and touch your partner and share your thoughts and the benefit of your life experiences and how you have grown over the years and are still growing. With ease your partner can return your touch and you may enter a world you've not known before. Can this happen with the partner you have had for years? Of course. Can it happen with someone new? Yes, if you believe it can.

If these are issues that concern you or on which you simply want advice, seek the help of a therapist or doctor who, you may be surprised to learn, has dealt with these kinds of matters many times and will not be surprised by what you have to say. Like doctors, therapists are sworn to confidentiality, which protects you and is in their own self-interest. So going to a therapist is strongly advised if you feel that your sex life could be better.

Also, the National Institute on Aging Information Center can help by sending you free publications. Contact the Center at P.O. Box 8057, Gaithersburg, MD 20898-8057 or call, toll-free, 800-222-2225. More importantly, listen to your own mind and body and do what makes you comfortable—or even excited.

Sleep Deprivation

Plenty of anecdotal evidence suggests that sleep deprivation is the result of changing sleep patterns as we age. Sleep that is not refreshing can keep your body from the natural healing and muscle rejuvenation that happens while you sleep. And it can spoil your mood during waking hours.

According to the National Institute on Aging (NIA) Fact Sheet entitled "A Good Night's Sleep":

> "The normal sleep cycle consists of two different kinds of sleep—REM (rapid eye movement or dreaming sleep) and non-REM (quiet sleep). Everyone has about four or five cycles of REM and non-REM sleep a night. For older persons, the amount of time spent in the deepest stages of non-REM sleep decreases. This may explain why older people are thought of as light sleepers."

Insomnia is a common complaint among the elderly. This occurs when it takes a person 35 to 40 minutes to fall asleep, or when someone wakes up often or wakes up early and isn't able to get back to sleep. Sometimes this is coupled with sleep apnea, literally when breathing stops for up to two minutes many times during the night (either due to "central sleep apnea," when respiratory muscles pause, or "obstructive" sleep apnea, when there is a blockage to the flow of air through the neck passage). The sleeper is totally unaware of the apnea.

There are over-the-counter drugs to help with insomnia, but it's a good idea to ask a physician's advice. There are a number of legitimate sleeping aids that can keep sleepers off their backs—a factor that contributes to apnea. Or there are medications—even surgery—to help with apnea.

In the same general area, there is another disorder known as "nocturnal myoclonus," when legs twitch during sleep, causing momentary waking. The cause of these movements is not known, and there is no cure, but mild leg exercises may help.

But getting a good night's sleep, says the NIA, "can make a big difference in your quality of life." Here are their nine suggestions for a good night's sleep:

- Follow a regular schedule (go to sleep and get up at the same time each day. (While there is no set number of hours to suit everybody, the normal range is seven to eight hours of sleep a night).
- Try to exercise regularly (two to four hours before bedtime, so there is sufficient time for relaxation before sleep).
- Expose yourself to natural light in the afternoon (this helps your internal "sleep clock").
- Watch your diet, avoid caffeine late in the day, and, if you snack, a glass of warm milk before bed will help.
- If you want to sleep well, don't smoke or drink alcohol (stimulants will keep you awake).
- Feel secure and comfortable. Lock all doors, in-

stall smoke alarms, keep a lamp nearby—or have remote control lighting—and keep a telephone by your bed. Sleep in a darkened and well-ventilated room.

- If you need to get up during the night, don't turn on overhead lights. Use small nightlights for navigating—and don't look at the time.
- Use your bedroom only for sleeping. Give yourself about 15 minutes to fall asleep; if you're still awake, get up, go to another room, and come back when you feel sleepy again.
- Try not to worry about your sleep. You might even want to play mental games or think about something you like or look forward to.

For More Information...

<u>General Information:</u>
A to Zzzz Guide to Better Sleep
Better Sleep Council
P.O. Box 13
Washington, D.C. 20044
E-Mail: <u>erinhill@ogilvypr.com</u>

<u>Sleep Disorders:</u>
The Association of Professional Sleep Societies
604 Second Street, SW
Rochester, MN 55902
703-683-8371

Or order *The Sleep Book*, published by AARP, 1909 K Street, N.W., Washington, DC 20049 (discounts for members).

Stroke

The Good News: Stroke can be prevented in many cases. In fact, the death rate from stroke has been cut in half in the past 30 years, due to Americans' improved health habits and the development of new diagnostic tests and treatments.

The Bad News: Stroke is the leading cause of long-term disability (American Heart Association, *Older Americans and Cardiovascular Diseases: Biostatistical Fact Sheets*, 1999: http://www.americanheart.org/statistics/biostats/biool.htm) and the third leading cause of death in the United States (*Deaths: Final Data for 1997*, National Vital Statistics Reports, Vol. 47, No. 19, National Center for Health Statistics, 1999). Three-quarters of those who have stroke in any year are over 65, and almost 90 percent of the deaths from stroke are in the over-65 age group. After age 55, the incidence of stroke doubles each decade.

According to the National Heart, Lung and Blood Institute:

> "A stroke is a sudden disruption in the flow of blood to an area of the brain. Deprived of blood, the affected brain cells either become damaged or die. While cell damage can often be repaired and the lost function regained, the death of brain cells is permanent and results in disability."

There are three types of strokes: thrombotic (the most common), in which fatty deposits build up in the arteries that supply blood to the brain, causing blockage; embolic, when a blood clot in an artery travels to the brain; and hemorrhagic, when a blood vessel in the brain bursts.

For More Information...

On the treatment and rehabilitation of strokes,
call a local teaching hospital or contact:

The American Heart Association
7320 Greenville Avenue
Dallas, TX 75231
800-AHA-USA1

A stroke requires hospitalization for immediate evaluation and treatment. A stroke can last minutes or hours; thus, if the patient is transferred to the hospital, often doctors can prevent blood clots from enlarging and causing further damage to the brain. The hospital staff usually conducts one or more of several tests: an electrocardiogram to measure electrical activity of the heart, an electroencephalogram to measure nerve cell activity in the brain, a CAT Scan to provide a three-dimensional picture, and an MRI to show the location of a blockage. In addition, the staff may administer anticoagulant drugs to arrest blockages.

However, you are your own best first line of defense against stroke:

- Control your blood pressure by having it checked regularly and, if it's too high, take steps to lower it (see "Blood Pressure/Hypertension," Page 224).
- If you are a smoker, STOP!
- Lower the fat content, saturated fatty acid, and cholesterol in your diet.

- Exercise regularly (exercise strengthens the heart).
- Control diabetes, if you have it (see "Diabetes," Page 242).
- Promptly report warning signs to your doctor (people experience "little strokes" [transient ischemic strokes], the clearest sign that a major stroke may be waiting in the wings).

To Get Answers to Your Questions

The National Institute of Neurological Disorders and Stroke (NINDS)
Information Office
Bldg. 31, Room 8A06
Bethesda, MD 20892
800-352-9424

The National Stroke Association
300 East Hampton Avenue, Suite 240
Englewood, CO 80110
800-367-1990

The conditions that can lead to a stroke are high blood pressure, arteriosclerosis, heart disease (see "Heart Disease," Page 254), diabetes, smoking, and being overweight.

Rehabilitation from a stroke can take weeks, months, or years. Physical therapy can strengthen muscles and improve balance. Speech and language therapy and occupational therapy can improve hand-eye coordination, which is necessary for daily tasks.

APPENDIX B

An Explanation of Government Health Care Programs

Medicare, Supplemental Insurance
Long-term Care Insurance
Medicaid ("MediCal" in California)

To many people, the terms *Medicare* and *Medicaid* connote complexity and confusion, but if you think of them simply as government-financed health insurance programs, perhaps the idea will be less daunting. *Government-financed* means that money comes either from federal and state general funds (supported by taxes) or from the Medicare Trust Fund (supported by premium deductions withheld as part of an employee's payroll).

Medicare insures Americans over 65 (and the disabled).

Medicaid (MediCal) insures eligible needy families with low incomes.

When Congress enacted these two programs in 1965, it marked the close of a debate that had started as early as 1915—a debate that had lasted through two world wars, the Depression, the New Deal and the Fair Deal, and the conflict in Korea. And all the while, America witnessed exponential growth in its industrial economy. It was part of President Lyndon Johnson's "Great Society," the culmination of debate on, and the enactment of, social concepts that seem today to have been a part of the national fabric forever; yet they came into being just under four decades ago.

Amendments and refinements made Medicare and Medicaid stand-alone programs in 1977 and gave them their own manager: The Health Care Financing Administration (HCFA), a major division of the U.S. Department of Health and Human Services.

While neither Medicare nor Medicaid covers the costs of every illness or condition, they do cover major health care needs and many minor ones. People who want or need greater coverage can buy, through health insurers, supplemental insurance that will help pay for the things that Medicare doesn't. (More on that later in this section.)

That leaves Americans who are neither over 65 nor low income (defined by a percentage of the "poverty level," which is a set limit, revised periodically, of income for individuals and couples). How are they covered?

The vast majority of the people in this category are employed and receive health insurance coverage as an employment benefit through private health insurers. Premiums are usually shared by employers and employees. Employers, acting as groups (sometimes even small businesses are allowed to ban together), can negotiate better premium rates by acting together. There is enough competition among private health insurers that these negotiations are meaningful in keeping premium costs from being higher.

But what about those who are not 65 or poor, and either not employed or employed by a business that doesn't offer health insurance as a benefit? These people are called the uninsured, or the underinsured in the case of an employer who offers only the most basic protection. And, because there is a growing gap between categories of relative wealth and lack of wealth in America, the number of uninsured and underinsured continues to grow. Ten years ago the U.S. Senate Committee on Health and Human Resources estimated that it would take an investment of $36 billion to cover this group; it would be even more today.

Health care in the United States is not cheap. In 1996 we passed the $1 trillion mark, and the figure is climbing. Today, with health care inflation (measured by what is called the "hospital market basket") running once again into double digits (far ahead of the Consumer Price Index), it should be clear that consumer demand for quality care is not diminishing. In fact, with the continuing growth of our older population, demand will certainly increase.

At the March, 2000, annual meeting of the American Society on Aging, renowned professor and author Theodore Roszak suggested that, while most people believe America is passing from an industrial economy to one based on information technology, we are becoming an economy based on health care. We spend nearly 14 percent of our gross domestic product on health care (or about $4,000 per person for every one of the more than 275 million people in the nation.

Thus, we have a health care system in the United States that is partially funded by the government (Medicare and Medicaid), partially funded by private health insurers) and partially not insured at all.

Remember that the federal government requires that for a hospital to be licensed and receive federal funds under Medicare and Medicaid, it must agree to treat anyone who comes to its emergency room. This often means that hospitals cannot recover costs for treating patients who need emergency care and cannot pay for it. This begs the question of what is called "cost shifts," whereby hospitals shift those costs, if they can, to other paying patients by what they charge them.

Health care coverage in this country has been debated for a century and the new century will be no different. Some people argue for a national health care system in which everyone is covered by government-financed insurance. There is a wide variety of proposals along these lines, but invariably they have run into opposition on two grounds: the huge price tag, and fear of an even bigger government bureaucracy.

Opponents often point to nations like Canada, Belgium, and England, which have their own varieties of national health care. By demonstrating some of the quality of care experiences in those systems, and by showing what illnesses and conditions are not covered, those opponents have prevailed to date. This still leaves a stalemate when it comes to the uninsured and the underinsured.

Medicare Coverage

Medicare has three parts: A, B, and C. The different parts simply indicate to whom payment is made. Part A reimburses hospitals and other health care institutions. Part B pays doctors and qualified health care professionals. And Part C, called "Medicare + Choice," provides an option for beneficiaries who are already covered under Parts A and B. Under Part C, people can choose services provided by managed care (Health Maintenance Organizations [HMOs], Provider-Sponsored Organizations [PSOs], Preferred Provider Organizations [PPOs]), certain private fee-for-service plans that accept Medicare rates, and medical savings account plans (usually carrying a high deductible).

Part A is hospital insurance that covers five main types of institutions:

- **Inpatient Hospital Care:** Virtually all hospital costs (semiprivate room) including surgery, medications, intensive care, nursing, tests and X-rays, in-patient rehabilitation, and medical supplies. There is an initial deductible, then 100 percent coverage for 60 days; however, a co-payment is required after 60 days up to the maximum time allowed under the benefit.

- **Skilled Nursing Facility:** If you've been in the hospital for three or more days and you require skilled nursing care within 30 days of your release, the same costs that are covered for in-patient hospital care are covered, but only for a maximum of 100 days (with a co-payment starting on the 21st day). Note that there is no coverage if the patient does not require *skilled* nursing care.

NOTE: Many people think that Medicare covers the cost of skilled nursing facility (nursing home) care. Generally, it does not! It does so *only* to the extent outlined above. (See the discussion on long-term care insurance, Page 294.)

- **Home Health Agency (HHA):** This includes a home health aide. Care may be furnished by a home health agency and is intermittent or part-time. There must be a plan of treatment that is periodically reviewed by a physician, but there is no deductible, co-payment, or time limitation. Some medical equipment is covered, but the patient must pay 20 percent of the cost.
- **Hospice Care:** For patients who choose, hospice care is covered in lieu of hospital care. Patients must be terminally ill, judged by physicians to have a life expectancy of six months or less. All hospice services are covered, including pain relief, medical and social services, and physical therapy. If, during that time, a condition arises that is not related to the terminal illness, Medicare will pay for the services required by that condition. There are no deductibles, but there is a small co-payment for drugs and in-patient respite care.

- **Programs of All-Inclusive Care for the Elderly (PACE):** This coverage is coupled with Medicaid and is an alternative to institutional care for people over 55 who require a nursing facility level of care and who meet eligibility requirements. PACE programs operate in only a limited number of areas of the country.

Services that are *not* covered under Medicare include long-term nursing care (custodial care), dentures and dental care, eyeglasses, hearing aids, and most prescription drugs. It is the debate over possible coverage of prescription drugs that has occupied national attention, as well it should. Medicare D

Today three-fourths of Medicare beneficiaries have chronic health problems requiring prescription drugs. The good news is that such drugs have been discovered and are available. They are the result of breakthroughs in Alzheimer's and Parkinson's Disease, diabetes, heart disease, and other chronic illnesses. With these advances, there is more reliance on prescription drugs as contrasted to the invasive patient procedures of years ago that were the initial focus of Medicare legislation.

The bad news is that older adults on a fixed income must now spend more of their resources for prescription drugs than ever before. If you are among the 30 percent of all seniors with an income below $10,000, you may become part of the one in eight American seniors who has to choose between food and drugs. (Three-fourths of America's seniors have an annual income below $25,000.)

The charges for prescription drugs are whatever the market will bear. Drug manufacturers give large discounts to major purchasers, so if you are among the 30 percent of Medicare beneficiaries with no supplemental insurance (see the discussion on "supplemental insurance," below), the federal government (not being a volume purchaser) can't negotiate for you. Thus, you pay top dollar out of your own pocket.

Even supplemental health insurers have sharply scaled back benefits in recent years. But most of those with the lowest incomes are also the ones who can't afford supplemental insurance, yet they are the ones forced to pay the going price for prescription drugs.

Increasingly higher prices are attributed in part to the costs of research into newer drugs to match obvious demand and the lengthy stretch of time it takes to obtain approvals from the Food and Drug Administration (FDA). Not many of us would deny the role of the FDA in ensuring efficacy and safety (especially if we recall the days before such government guarantees were ordered by Congress), but it adds to the expense. And, there is greater demand by consumers in what some call a health care economy in which the population of older adults is growing rapidly.

Former President Clinton called for coverage for almost all those covered by Medicare, but those more concerned about overall costs are saying that such coverage for prescription drugs should be for the poor alone at lesser cost. This debate will likely continue. Even with unprecedented budget surpluses, there is plenty of political competition for those funds (the long-term solvency of Medicare and Social Security, paying down the

National Debt, the new (2001) major tax cut, and a host of other worthy proposals).

Look for some action now that the tax cut of 2001 is behind us. For too many Americans, this issue has become crucial. The question is not *whether* an expansion of Medicare to cover prescription drugs will be enacted by Congress, but *when* and to what extent.

Supplemental Insurance

The list of what Medicare provides may be impressive, but it should also be clear that the list has serious omissions and limitations. It would be a serious mistake to think that Medicare is a panacea that will cover you for all illnesses and conditions at all times and places from age 65 to the grave. It won't!

There must be some limitations on Medicare; otherwise, given the demand for health care in this country and the tremendous growth in the population over 65, the cost of Medicare would bankrupt the richest nation in the world. That doesn't mean you have to be let wanting, if you can afford the added premium.

Supplementary Medical Insurance (SMI), also colloquially called MediGap, is the government's version of supplementing Medicare coverage with a self-paying premium (minus the profit motive). It is usually cheaper than private insurance, but it provides less coverage on the average, and there may be more limitations, particularly as the demand for health care increases. People who are covered by Medicare can buy SMI, and almost 40 million people do. Almost nine out of every ten enrollees actually receive benefits, now approaching over $75 billion in the cost of services rendered.

SMI covers those non-hospital costs (Medicare covers the hospitals and institutions) that can skyrocket beyond Medicare's limits. Primarily that means physician services, clinical laboratory tests, durable medical equipment, most medical supplies, diagnostic tests, ambulance services, flu vaccinations, prescription drugs that cannot be self-administered, certain self-administered anti-cancer drugs, some therapy services, outpatient hospital services, ambulatory surgical centers, and home health agency services. There are other medical services that are subject to deductibles, maximum approved amounts, or higher cost-sharing.

In addition, there are a myriad of private and group supplemental policies that offer these same benefits, and more. Competition for your business is keen; be a good shopper. Do comparisons of costs and benefits. Chart the differences of all vendors, even respected groups, and ask advice before you buy.

Long-term Care Insurance

Long-term care insurance really means insurance to cover the costs of being in a skilled nursing facility (nursing home). That's not the meaning of long-term care, of course, and one day the definition may change. The "care" that is "long-term," more and more, is being done in the home and the community and does not involve being in a nursing home.

Still, nomenclature aside, if you need care in a nursing home, you and your family will be thankful that the costs were covered by insurance, if you can afford the premiums. The alternative is that you "spend down" your income and your assets to become eligible for

Medicaid, which will then pay your costs. This leaves you totally dependent on the government, robs you of your independence and dignity, and short-changes your family.

But long-term care insurance is not cheap. The very best premiums for reasonable coverage today are negotiated group plans, which feature premiums that do not escalate with age even though they are based on your age at time of purchase. The younger you are, the lower the premium, but the longer you have to pay it. Perhaps the most accomplished group plan for long-term care insurance today is the California Public Employees Retirement System (CALPERS). For a husband and wife, aged 60 and 50, respectively, in 1998, the combined premium was $184 per month. That rate is locked-in. That's $2,208 a year.

But just think! It will take this couple 20 years of premiums ($44,160) to insure against what it would cost for a little more than one year for both of them in a nursing home, which costs $3,000-a-month, or $72,000-a-year! Is the insurance worth it? Of course! But having the money to afford it may be another matter.

That's why long-term care insurance premiums must become more affordable. As more people see the sense in having this type of insurance, the actuarial base will get bigger, competition among insurers will increase, and the quality of the coverage and the premiums will improve. Employers and employee unions need to take note!

Medicaid ("MediCal" in California) Coverage

Medicaid, originally enacted at the same time as

Medicare, serves needy families with low incomes. But not all those who are poor qualify; there are other criteria. In fact, eligibility varies from state to state. Almost 40 million people (of our population of more than 275 million) are receivers of services under Medicaid. Annual expenditures top $200 billion (federal and state funds) and are projected to reach $255 billion by 2003.

Whereas Medicare is totally funded by the federal government, Medicaid is generally half federal money and half state matching funds. The federal government provides broad guidelines through laws and regulations, but each state (including territories):

- Establishes its own eligibility standards,
- Determines the type, amount, duration, and scope of services,
- Sets the rate of payment for services, and
- Administers its own program.

This dual participation by federal and state governments ensures that neither level of government will over-commit the other financially and provides a partnership in accounting for wide differences among states (e.g. urbanized as contrasted to rural). But it also means that Medicaid is quite complex, with multiple standards of eligibility and services. It is probable, of course, that the same person who is eligible for Medicaid in one state may not be eligible in an adjacent state. Similarly, a health care service provided under Medicaid in one state may not be available next door.

At the same time, the federal government has set some basic Medicaid eligibility and coverage as a minimum. And, over the years, Congress has altered and added to this basic list, often causing complaints from the states who want the federal half of the costs but don't want to see Congress mandating changes that cost them additional appropriations.

The Medicaid "Categorically Needy" Congressionally Mandated Eligibility Groups

- People who meet the eligibility requirements for the former Aid To Families With Dependent Children (AFDC) that were in effect on July 16, 1996 when AFDC was replaced by Temporary Assistance for Needy Families (TANF), the centerpiece of the Welfare Reform Act.
- Children under age 6 whose family income is at or below 133 percent of the federal poverty level (FPL: a changing indicator barely into five figures).
- Pregnant women whose family is below 133 percent of FPL (services must be related to pregnancy, delivery, and postpartum care).
- Supplemental Security Income (a unit of the Social Security Act) recipients in most states.
- Recipients of adoption or foster care assistance under Title IV of the Social Security Act.
- People who may keep Medicaid eligibility for a period of time even as they are emerging from TANF by work earnings or nominally increased Social Security benefits.
- By 2002, all children under age 19 in families at or below the FPL.

Continued

In addition, there are several groups described as **"categorically related"** that may be included at state option for which the federal government will pay half. Chief among these are infants up to age 1 and pregnant women up to 185 percent of FPL, institutionalized individuals up to a "special income level" to be set by each state, and certain low-income aged, blind, and disabled adults.

States may also designate those who are **"medically needy"** (above the FPL, but still low income) but this often requires people to "spend down" to be eligible.

In the Balanced Budget Act of 1997 (BBA), Medicaid was expanded again—this time to benefit children who are part of the uninsured population. The Children's Health Insurance Program (CHIP) encouraged states to develop programs that would cover as many uninsured children as possible, with the federal government agreeing to pick up half the tab. One of the hallmarks of this expansion is a vastly simplified eligibility application, which is intended to remove a paperwork barrier that often inhibits participation in other social and health care government programs.

Federally Mandated Scope of Medicaid Services

- Inpatient and outpatient hospital services
- Prenatal care

- Vaccines for children
- Physician services
- Nursing facility services for people 21 or older
- Family planning services and supplies
- Rural health clinic services
- Home health care for persons otherwise eligible for skilled nursing services
- Laboratory tests and X-rays
- Pediatric, nurse practitioner, and midwife services
- Early and periodic screening, diagnostic, and treatment services for children under 21

There are 34 **optional services** that states can elect to provide and still receive federal financial participation. Chief among these are:
- diagnostic and clinic services,
- intermediate care for the mentally retarded,
- prescription drugs and prosthetic devices,
- eyeglasses,
- rehabilitation and physical therapy,
- home and community-based care to certain persons with chronic impairments, and
- transportation services.

In BBA, Congress also expanded Medicaid to include the Programs of All-Inclusive Care for the Elderly (PACE). PACE is an alternative for those over 55 who require a "nursing facility level of care." PACE puts together a team approach to health care and social services that helps each participant retain independence and quality of life.

It is not inexpensive (which is why it is limited to a small number of locations), but it may be possible to prove in time that PACE is not as expensive as skilled nursing homes. PACE can also mobilize care provided directly in private homes, day health centers, hospitals, and nursing homes. PACE was started as a pilot program in San Francisco more than 20 years ago and has now proven itself to the point of this expansion.

At the same time, it should be understood that the Medicaid program has had a more rapid growth in expenditures than Medicare. The type of person utilizing Medicaid, and the average cost, demonstrate why. Medicaid was originally enacted to care for poor families and their children who were tied to welfare eligibility. Today more than 45 percent of the cost of those in nursing homes or using home health services (the most rapidly growing service provider category) is paid for by Medicaid. Another way to view this impact is to note that, while children account for 46 percent of Medicaid's patients, they cost only $1,000 per child per year, whereas the average annual cost of an adult is $3,400.

The major reasons for cost increases are:
- Expanded coverage and utilization mandated by Congress,
- Congress' enactment of subsidies to hospitals providing care for uninsured indigents, called disproportionate share,
- Huge increases in very old and disabled persons requiring extensive acute or long-term care,
- Technological advances that can be costly in terms of patient care, and
- Health care inflation that continually runs sub-

stantially ahead of general inflation (the U.S. Consumer Price Index).

Medicare and Medicaid Together

People who are eligible for Medicare, having reached age 65, and who are also eligible for Medicaid, depending on the state or territory they live in, are called "dually eligible." This works to ensure that the frail elderly who are low income do not slip between the cracks.

In these cases the Medicaid program acts as a supplement to Medicare. Essentially, it means that dually eligible patients receive the benefits of Medicare and whatever benefits are offered by the state in which they live. Examples might include nursing facility care beyond that provided by Medicare, some prescription drugs, eyeglasses, and hearing aids.

Notwithstanding state eligibility standards, Congress has designated certain low-income people to be covered. These are called Qualified Medicare Beneficiaries (QMBs), Special Low-Income Medicare Beneficiaries (SLMBs) and Qualified Disabled and Working Individuals (QDWIs). These designations refer to people who are measured against the federal poverty level and who are mandated to be covered wherever they live. In addition, Congress has provided that people in these groups have their premiums for Supplemental Medicare Insurance (SMI) paid for by federal funds

Health Care Reform

The Congressional plate is full of proposals to modify our health care system. From coverage for prescription drugs to solvency for the Medicare Trust Fund to coverage for the uninsured to the quality of managed care to enactment of a patient's bill of rights. Each of these topics directly affects the other, which is why it is difficult to achieve comprehensive reform. Federal and state constraints, however, include serious economic, social, and political factors—elements that have been present ever since the debates started in 1915.

This section on "Medicare, Supplemental Insurance, Long-term Care Insurance and Medicaid" is based on a monograph entitled, *Brief Summaries of Medicare and Medicaid, Title XVIII and Title XIX of the Social Security Act (July 31, 1998)*, prepared by Mary Onnis Waid, Social Science Research Analyst, Office of the Actuary, Health Care Financing Administration, U.S. Department of Health and Human Services.

For More Information...

AARP Public Policy Institute
601 E Street, NW
Washington, D.C. 20049
800-424-3410
web site www.aarp.org

National Committee to Preserve Social Security and Medicare
10 G Street, NE, #600
Washington, D.C. 20002
800-966-1935

Medicare Rights Center
1460 Broadway
New York, NY 10036
212-869-3850
web site: www.medicarerights.org
(ask for publications brochure)

The Urban Institute
2100 M Street, NW
Washington, D.C. 20037
202-833-7200
web site: www.urban.org
(public policy monographs)

American Society on Aging
833 Market Street, #511
San Francisco, CA 94103-1824
415-974-0300
(extensive library/research center)

Alliance for Aging Research
2021 K Street, NW, #305
Washington, D.C. 20006
202-293-2856

"Shaping the Future of Medicare"
by Karen Davis, April, 1998
The Commonwealth Fund
One East 75th Street
New York, NY 10021-2692
212-535-0400

Continued

"The Uninsured and Their Access to Health Care"
(July, 1998)
The Henry J. Kaiser Family Foundation
1450 G Street, NW, #250
Washington, DC 20005
202-347-5270
web site: www.kff.org

For a booklet explaining the "CalPERS LTC Program":

The California Long Term Care Partnership
Route W207, P.O. Box 5708
Hopkins, MN 55343-5708
800-908-9119

Office of Public Affairs, CalPERS
400 P Street
Sacramento, CA 95814
916-326-3036

APPENDIX C

A Resource Directory

Resources for older adults already abound at the national, state, and local levels. For years, particularly since the inception of Medicare and the Older Americans Act, a whole network has evolved throughout the country to provide information and choices of services.

Many think of these services as being available only to those who qualify by virtue of income or minority status. Not so! For example, if you wish a congregate meal at a senior center, all you need do is show up (or call for transportation, if you need it). If you need information on health conditions or long-term care planning or advice on legal issues, the people answering your call (often on a toll-free line) do not ask your income, status, or ethnicity. With appropriate information, you are better able to make choices.

Most national organizations have state and local counterparts. The U.S. Administration on Aging has its network of state units and local Area Agencies on Aging. AARP has state offices in every state; they, in turn, have local units of volunteers throughout the nation.

For those who want to embark on an information journey, here are some of the major national groups (both governmental and non-profit), divided into five categories: Two umbrella government units, followed by listings for General Information, Health-related Information, Diet and Fitness, and Long-term Care.

The two overarching government resource entities on matters relating to aging are:

The U.S. Administration on Aging

330 Independence Avenue, S.W.
Washington, D.C. 20201

Telephone Numbers:

800-677-1116 (The ELDERCARE LOCATOR; use this number to find services in your own locality)
(Web Site: www.ageinfo.org/elderloc/elderdb.html)
202-619-0724 (AoA's Main Number)
E-Mail: aoainfo@ban-gate.aoa.dhhs.gov
Web Site: http://www.aoa.gov

202-619-7501 (AoA's National Aging Information
Center [NAIC]—for technical information
and public inquiries),
E-Mail: aoainfo@aoa.gov or naic@aoa.gov
Web Site: www.aoa.gov/naic

"The Administration on Aging (AoA) is the federal focal point and advocacy agency for older persons. Under the Older Americans Act, the AoA works closely with its nationwide network of state and Area Agencies on Aging and service providers to plan, coordinate and develop community-level systems of services that help vulnerable older persons to remain in their own homes by providing supportive services and other programs." (AoA's Mission Statement)

The National Institute on Aging

Building 31, Room 5C27
31 Center Drive, MSC 2292
Bethesda, MD 20892-2292
301-496-1752
E-Mail: niainfo@access.digex.net
Web Site: www.nih.gov.nia

Information Clearinghouse: 800-222-2225 (toll-free)

"The National Institute on Aging (NIA), part of the National Institutes of Health, is the federal government's principal agency for conducting and supporting biomedical, social and behavioral research related to aging processes and the diseases and special problems of older people." (NIA's Mission Statement)

You can use these contacts to get information on almost any topic. If the answer is not readily available, then a number of other organizations may be able to provide more targeted information.

Resource Directory: General Information

National Association of State Units on Aging (NASUA)
1225 I Street, N.W.
Washington, D.C. 20005
202-898-2578
E-Mail: staff@nasua.org

NASUA is a national public interest organization that provides information, technical assistance, and professional development support to its members. NASUA works to promote social policy at the federal and state levels responsive to the needs of older Americans.

National Association of Area Agencies on Aging (N4A)
927 15th Street, N.W., Sixth Floor
Washington, D.C. 20005
202-296-8130
Web Site: www.n4a.org

N4A represents the interests of Area Agencies on Aging across the country.

American Association of Retired Persons (AARP)
601 E Street, N.W.
Washington, D.C. 20049
202-434-2277
Web Site: www.aarp.org

AARP is a nonprofit membership organization dedicated to helping older Americans achieve lives of independence, dignity, and purpose.

American Society on Aging (ASA)
833 Market Street, Suite 511
San Francisco, CA 94103
415-974-9600
E-Mail: info@asa.asaging.org   Web Site: www.asaging.org

ASA is a nonprofit membership organization that informs the public and health professionals about issues affecting the quality of life for older people and promotes innovative approaches to meet those needs.

Elderhostel
75 Federal Street
Boston, MA 02110-1941
617-426-7788
Web Site: www.elderhostel.org

Elderhostel is a nonprofit organization committed to being the preeminent provider of high-quality, affordable educational opportunities for older adults. Sharing new ideas, challenges, and experiences is rewarding in every season of life. Programs are held at colleges, universities, and other educational and cultural institutions throughout the U.S., Canada, and more than 70 countries overseas.

National Interfaith Coalition on Aging

(National Council on Aging)
409 3rd Street, S.W., Suite 200
Washington, D.C. 20024
202-479-1200
Web Site: www.ncoa.org

The National Interfaith Coalition on Aging, a program of the National Council on Aging (NCOA), includes representatives of the Roman Catholic, Jewish, Protestant, and Orthodox faiths and others concerned with religion and aging. The Coalition supports individuals and religious groups that serve older people.

Ethnic Groups

National Indian Council on Aging

10501 Montgomery Boulevard, N.E.
Albuquerque, NM 87111
505-292-1922 (fax)
Web Site: www.nicoa.org

NICOA, a nonprofit advocate for older American Indians and Alaskan Natives, is funded by the Administration on Aging and works to provide improved, comprehensive services to American Indian and Alaskan Native elders.

**National Resource Center on
Native American Aging**
P.O. Box 7090
Grand Forks, ND 58202-7090
800-896-7628
E-Mail: allery@badlands.nodak.edu
Web Site: www.und.nodak.edu/dept/nrcnaa

The National Resource Center on Native American Aging serves the older Native American population of the United States. The Center is committed to increasing the awareness of issues affecting American Indian, Alaskan Native, and Native Hawaiian elders and being a voice and advocate for their concerns. The Center provides education, training, technical assistance, and research.

National Asian Pacific Center on Aging
Melbourne Tower
1511 3rd Avenue, Suite 914
Seattle, WA 98101-1626
206-624-1221. Information Service: 800-336-2722
Web Site: www.nwlink.com/~scpnwan/articles/05-17-97/grant/html

The National Asian Pacific Center on Aging serves as the leading national advocacy organization committed to the dignity, well-being and quality of life of Asian Pacific Americans in their senior years.

National Hispanic Council on Aging
(Meeting the Special Concerns of Hispanic Older Women)
2713 Ontario Road, N.W.
Washington, D.C. 20009
E-Mail: nhcoa@worldnep.att.net
Web Site: www.incacorp.com/nhcoa

NHCOA is a private, nonprofit organization that works to promote the well-being of older Hispanics by sponsoring demonstration projects, publishing educational materials that are culturally and linguistically appropriate, hosting training institutes for people who work with older Hispanics (particularly women), and developing programs for Latino gerontology students.

National Association for Hispanic Elderly – Asociacion Nacional Por Personas Mayores
1452 West Temple Street, Suite 100
Los Angeles, CA 90026-1724
213-487-1922

The National Association for Hispanic Elderly works to ensure that older Hispanic citizens are included in all social service programs for older Americans through a system of regional offices that provide information about the needs and capabilities of older Hispanics to both private and public agencies.

Special Purpose

Brookdale Center on Aging
425 East 25th Street
New York, NY 10010
212-481-4426. Information Service: 800-647-8233
E-Mail: brookdale@shiva.hunter.cuny.edu
Web Site: www.brookdale.org
   The Brookdale Center on Aging of Hunter College offers professional training and support to those who provide services to older people, including up-to-date research and publications, such as The Senior Rights Reporter, *a quarterly journal.*

Generations Together
University Center for Social and Urban Research
University of Pittsburgh
121 University Place, Suite 300
Pittsburgh, PA 15260-5907
412-648-7150
E-Mail: mitchl@pitt.edu
Web Site: www.pitt.edu/~gti/
   Generations Together's programs place youth and elders together in a multitude of human service projects. These projects bring a unique dimension to human services because they join two populations in a common cause.

Resource Directory: Health

Agency for Health Care Policy and Research (AHCPR)
P.O. Box 8547
Silver Spring, MD 20907-8547
410-290-3684. Publications Clearinghouse: 800-358-9295
Web Site: www.ahcpr.gov

The Purpose of AHCPR is to enhance the quality, appropriateness, and effectiveness of health care services and to improve access to that care.

Alzheimer's Association
919 North Michigan Avenue, Suite 1000
Chicago, IL 60611
312-335-8700. Information & Referral: 800-272-3900
Web Site: www.alz.org

The Alzheimer's Association is a voluntary organization that sponsors public education programs and offers supportive services to patients and families who are coping with Alzheimer's Disease. A 24-hour toll-free hot line (above) provides information about Alzheimer's Disease and links families with local chapters that are familiar with community resources and can offer practical suggestions for daily living. The Association also funds research to find a cure for Alzheimer's Disease.

American Cancer Society
2525 Ridge Point Drive, Suite 100
Austin, TX 78745
404/320-3333. Cancer Response System: 800-227-2345
Web Site: www. cancer.org/frames.html

The American Cancer Society is a national, community-based volunteer health organization whose mission is to eliminate cancer as a major health problem by promoting its prevention. ACS seeks to diminish patients' suffering through research, education, advocacy, and patient services. The Society supports medical and scientific research in all aspects of cancer and provides education to inform the public about various forms of the disease, as well as issues of early detection, risk reduction, and prevention. Local ACS units sponsor a wide range of services for cancer patients and their families, including self-help groups, transportation programs, and limited financial aid.

American Diabetes Association
1660 Duke Street
Alexandria, VA 22314
703-549-1500 . Information Service: 800-342-2383
Web Site: www.diabetes.org

The mission of the American Diabetes Association is to prevent and cure diabetes and to improve the lives of all people affected by diabetes. The Association works to educate the public to recognize the warning signs of diabetes and to realize the importance of prompt treatment. It has a nationwide system of local chapters.

American Foundation for the Blind
11 Penn Plaza, Suite 300
New York, NY 10001
212-502-7777. Information Service: 800-232-5463
Web Site: www.terraquest.com/highsights/afb/afbintro.html

The American Foundation for the Blind is a national, nonprofit organization whose mission is to enable people who are blind or visually impaired to achieve equality of access and opportunity that will ensure freedom of choice in their lives. The Foundation offers expertise in education, employment, aging, technology, and access to agencies, schools, other organizations, and professionals in the field of blindness.

American Heart Association
7272 Greenville Avenue
Dallas, TX 75231
Heart and Stroke Information: 800-242-8721
Web Site: www.americanheart.org

The American Heart Association is a nonprofit, voluntary health organization, funded by private contributions, with a mission to reduce disability and death from cardiovascular diseases and stroke. These include heart attack, stroke (brain attack), and related disorders. (Cardiovascular diseases are the nation's number one killer.) The Association's mission also includes providing reliable information to the American public on prevention and treatment of heart disease and stroke. It has about 2,000 state and metropolitan affiliates, divisions, and branches throughout the nation.

Arthritis Foundation
1330 West Peachtree Street
Atlanta, GA 30309
404-872-7100. Information Service: 800-283-7800
Web Site: www.arthritis.org

The Arthritis Foundation is a nonprofit, volunteer organization that supports research to find a cure for, and ways to prevent, all forms of arthritis. It also seeks to improve the

quality of life for people with arthritis. The Foundation's na-
tionwide chapters offer health education programs in local
communities, including arthritis self-help courses, aquatic
programs, exercise programs, support groups, and public fo-
rums.

National AIDS Hotline
P.O. Box 13827
Research Triangle Park, NC 27709
919-361-8400
Web Site: www.ashastd.org/nah/nah.html
The National AIDS Hotline, a service of the Centers for
Disease Control and Prevention, is the primary HIV/AIDS
information, education, and referral service for the United
States:
Hotline: 800-342-2437 (English), 800-344-7432 (Span-
ish), 800-243-7889 (TTY)

National Association of the Deaf
814 Thayer Avenue
Silver Spring, MD 20910
301-587-1791
E-Mail: nadhq@juno.com
Web Site: www.nad.org
The mission of the National Association of the Deaf is to
assure that a comprehensive coordinated system of service is
accessible to Americans who are deaf and hard of hearing,
enabling them to achieve their maximum potential through
increased independence, productivity, and integration. As-
sociation programs include a youth leadership camp, a legal
defense fund, Interpreter and Sign Language Interpreter cer-
tification, and biannual conventions.

National Cancer Institute
Office of Cancer Communications
Building 31, Room 10A07
31 Center Drive MSC 2580
Bethesda, MD 20892-2580
301/496-5583. Information Service: 800-422-6237
Web Site: http://rex.nci.nih.gov

The National Cancer Institute, part of the National Institutes of Health, is the federal government's principle agency for funding cancer research and for distributing information about cancer to health professionals and the public. One of NCI's priorities is a national education initiative targeting people age 65 and older and the health professionals who treat them.

National Council on Alcoholism and Drug Dependence
12 West 21st Street, 7th Floor
New York, NY 10010
212-206-6770 . Information Service: 800-622-2255 or 800-475-4673
E-Mail: national@ncadd.org
Web Site: www.ncadd.org

NCADD is a private, nonprofit organization that works to educate the public about the prevention and treatment of alcoholism and drug dependence and acts as an advocate on behalf of alcoholics, other addicted persons, and their families. The Council has a network of local chapters around the country.

National Multiple Sclerosis Society
733 3rd Avenue, Sixth Floor
New York, NY 10017
212-986-3240. Information Service: 800-344-4867
E-Mail: nat@nmss.org
Web Site: www.nmss.org

NMSS is a nonprofit organization dedicated to the prevention, treatment, and cure of multiple sclerosis and to the improved quality of life for people with MS and their families. The Society has local chapters nationwide that engage in educational programs, information and referral, counseling, and public policy advocacy.

National Osteoporosis Foundation
1150 17th Street, N.W., Suite 500
Washington, D.C. 20036-4603
202-223-2226
Web Site: www.nof.org

The National Osteoporosis Foundation is a volunteer health agency dedicated to reducing osteoporosis, a condition seen most often in older women. Osteoporosis causes bone density to decrease, which produces weakness throughout the skeleton and leads to an increased risk of fractures.

National Stroke Association
96 Inverness Drive East, Suite I
Englewood, CO 80112-5112
303-649-9299
Web Site: www.stroke.org

The National Stroke Association provides information to the public and health professionals about strokes and offers supportive services to stroke survivors and their families.

Self-Help for Hard of Hearing People, Inc.
7910 Woodmont Avenue, Suite 1200
Bethesda, MD 20814
301-657-2248, 301-657-2249 (TTY)
Web Site: www.shhh.org

SHHH seeks to make mainstream society more accessible to people who are hard of hearing and to improve the quality of life of hard of hearing people through education, advocacy, and self-help.

The Skin Cancer Foundation
245 5th Avenue
New York, NY 10016
212-725-5176. Information Service: 800-754-6490
E-Mail: info@skincancer.org
Web Site: www.skincancer.org

The Skin Cancer Foundation is a nonprofit public information organization that stresses early detection/treatment of skin cancer.

Resource Directory: Diet and Fitness

American Dietetic Association
216 West Jackson Boulevard
Chicago, IL 60606-6995
312/899-0040. Publications Service: 800-745-0775.
Consumer Hotline: 800-366-1655
Web Site: www.eatright.org

The American Dietetic Association is a professional society of dieticians who work in health care settings, schools, day care centers, business and industry, and Area Agencies on Aging. Registered dieticians provide expertise on nutrition.

Food and Nutrition Information Center
National Agriculture Library Building, Room 304
U.S. Department of Agriculture
Bethesda, MD 20705-2351
301-504-5719
E-Mail: fnic@nalusda.gov
Web Site: www.nalusda.gov/fnic
The Food and Nutrition Information Center, a service of the federal government, provides information to professionals and the public on human nutrition, food service management, and food technology.

Meals on Wheels Association of America
1414 Prince Street, Suite 202
Alexandria, VA 22314
703-548-5558
E-Mail: mowaa@tbg.dgsys.com
Web Site: www.projectmeal.org
MOWAA is the oldest organization in the United States representing those who provide meals to people in need. The Association provides education, training, and development opportunities, enabling members to provide quality nutrition services and programs. MOWAA ensures that older Americans have access to nutritious meals by offering training and technical assistance to those who plan and conduct congregate and home-delivered meal programs throughout the nation.

**National Policy/Resource Center
on Nutrition and Aging**
Florida International University
University Park, OE200
Miami, FL 33199
305-348-1517
E-Mail: nutrelder@solix.fiu.edu
Web Site: www.fiu.edu/~nutreldr

The National Center, working with the Administration on Aging, aims to improve the nutritional status of older Americans by focusing on information dissemination.

National Senior Sports Association
83 Princeton Avenue
Hopewell, NJ 08525
609-466-0022. Information Service: 800-282-6772
or 800-752-9718
Web Site: www.amgolftour.com

The National Senior Sports Association is a membership organization for men and women over 50 who enjoy golf/travel.

President's Council on Physical Fitness and Sports
200 Independence Avenue, S.W., Suite 738-H
Washington, D.C. 20201
202-690-9000
Web Site: www.hhs.gov/progorg/ophs/pcpfs.htm

The Council distributes information to the public about the health-related benefits of regular exercise.

American Alliance for Health,
Physical Education, Recreation and Dance
1900 Association Drive
Reston, VA 20191
703-476-3400. Information Service: 800-213-7193
E-Mail: webmaster@aahperd.org
Web Site: www.aahperd.org
  AAHPERD is an organization of professionals supporting those involved in phys ed, dance and a healthy lifestyle.

Resource Directory: Long-Term Care

Aging Network Services
4400 East-West Highway, Suite 907
Bethesda, MD 20814
301-657-4329
Web Site: www.agingnets.com/
  Aging Network Services is a nationwide, for-profit network of private-practice geriatric social workers serving as care managers for older parents. The Network provides assessment, guidance and recommendations, arrangement for home care services, selection of placements, psychotherapy, and consultation.

Assisted Living Federation of America
10300 Eaton Place, Suite 400
Fairfax, VA 22031
703-691-8100
Web Site: www.alfa.org

ALFA is a national nonprofit trade association dedicated to enhancing the quality of life in assisted living residences and representing the interests of the assisted living industry.

National Association of Home Care
Foundation for Hospice and Home Care
228 7th Street, N.E.
Washington, D.C. 20003
202-547-7424
Web Site: www.nahc.org

The Association is a professional organization that represents a variety of agencies providing home care services, including home health agencies, hospice programs, and homemaker/home health aid agencies.

The Foundation promotes hospice and home care, establishes responsible standards of care, develops programs to ensure the proper preparation of caregivers, educates the public, and conducts research on aging, health and social policies.

The Foundation also maintains a Directory of Accredited or Approved Home Care Aides Services, *which is updated twice annually. It publishes, and distributes free, consumer guides on home care and hospice care.*

National Citizens' Coalition for Nursing Home Reform/National Long Term Care Ombudsman Resource Center
1424 16th Street, N.W., Suite 202
Washington, D.C. 20036-2211
E-Mail: nccnhrl@erols.com
Web Site: www.nccnhr.org

The Coalition defines and achieves quality for people with long-term care needs through informed, empowered consumers; effective citizens groups and ombudsman programs; promotion of best practices in care delivery; public policy responsive to consumer needs; and enforcement of consumer-directed health and living standards. The Coalition has state affiliates nationwide; in California the affiliate, California Advocates for Nursing Home Reform (CANHR), publishes a list of California nursing homes, by county, with relevant commentary and facts, on its web site: www.cahnr.org

The Ombudsman Resource Center supports the ongoing development and operation of the state's long-term care ombudsman programs. It is operated by the Coalition in collaboration with the National Association of State Units on Aging (NASUA).

National Long Term Care Resource Center
Institute for Health Services Research
University of Minnesota School of Public Health
420 Delaware Street, Box 197 Mayo
Minneapolis, MN 55455
612-624-5171
Web Site: www.hsr.umn.edu/

The Center, a collaboration between the University of Minnesota Institute for Health Services Research and the National Academy of State Health Policy, assists the aging network to develop, administer, monitor, and refine community-based long-term care systems reform.

The Center's three focal points are: ethics and decision-making; links between long-term care and acute care, rehabilitation, and health care reform; and assessment and case management (emphasizing clinical applications).

National Resource and Policy Center on Housing and Long Term Care

Andrus Gerontology Center
University of Southern California
Los Angeles, CA 90089-0191
213-740-1364
E-Mail: hmap@usc.edu
Web Site: www.usc.edu/go/hmap

The Center—in partnership with N4A, Brandeis University and the National Association of Housing and Redevelopment Officials—works to make housing an integral part of long-term care.

National Resource and Policy Center on Rural Long Term Care

Center on Aging, University of Kansas Medical Center
3901 Rainbow Boulevard
Kansas City, KS 66160-7117
913-588-1636
Web Site: www.kumc.edu/instruction/medicine/NRPC

The Center focuses on improving the availability of community-based long-term care in rural areas for the elderly and the disabled.

National Resource Center on Long Term Care

(National Association of State Units on Aging)
1225 I Street, N.W., Suite 725
Washington, D.C. 20005
202-898-2578 AgeNet Electronic Bulletin Board: 202-898-4794

The Center concentrates on improvement and enhancement of community-based care and emphasizes consumer involvement.

**National Resource Center: Diversity
and Long Term Care**
Heller School, Institute for Health Policy, Brandeis University
P.O. Box 9110
Waltham, MA 02254-9110
781-736-3930. Information Service: 800-456-9966
Jointly operated by Brandeis and San Diego State University, the Center concentrates on diversity issues: resource distribution, infrastructure, care strategies, and consumer roles and choices.

Resource Directory: Advocacy

The term *advocacy* takes on two meanings, both related to older adults, particularly the frail elderly, but directed at different audiences. *Webster's New World Dictionary* says that advocacy is "pleading another's cause or in support of something."

In the setting of a nursing home, an ombudsman may plead the cause of the patient by calling attention to some unmet need, particularly when the patient can't communicate. In that sense, the audience is the nursing home staff, and the ombudsman is being the patient's "advocate." In one way or another, directly or indirectly, through thousands of staff and volunteers, every organization listed in this directory—and many not listed for lack of space—are advocates for individual seniors and elderly and those with disabilities.

Some organizations are at the forefront of the other type of advocacy—public policy and funding issues. Their advocacy is simultaneously at the federal, state, and local levels, mostly with government entities but often with private corporations and small business. In this case, because the audience is broad, the advocacy is "…in support of something" (in other words, lobbying or, to phrase it more delicately, legislative advocacy).

For example, organizations representing professionals in the field of aging at the national level, such as the National Association of State Units on Aging (NASUA) and the National Association of Area Agencies on Aging (N4A) [both described on Page 308], testify before congressional committees and advocate the views of their members to officials in the executive branch of government.

AARP (also Page 308), because it is a private membership organization, can be more aggressive. It employs a staff whose sole purpose is to advocate on policy issues and for more funding for programs relating to aging. The Committee to Preserve Social Security and Medicare is similar in its advocacy.

By far, the most aggressive advocates, as organizations, are those that have a reform agenda. There can even be an element of anger and blame in the views of reformers because they see neglect or wrongdoing that, to them, is an outrage.

This does not mean that these groups do not perform constructive services, as well as advocacy. One major example is the National Citizen's Coalition for Nursing Home Reform (see Page 324) with the "reform" agenda right in its title; yet NCCNHR also performs a vital service of research and training staff and volunteers in the field as ombudsmen through its National Long Term Care Ombudsman Resource Center.

Reformers are vocal and understandably consumer oriented. When they are joined by more mainstream voices, action is virtually certain. That was the case recently in California where the California Advocates for Nursing Home Reform (CANHR) banded together, albeit with hesitation, with the California unit of AARP to convince the governor to sponsor reform legislation that he previously vetoed.

Other organizations at the forefront of public policy advocacy in an aggressive way are:

Gray Panthers
733 15th Street, N.W., Suite 437
Washington, D.C. 20005
202-737-6637. Information Service: 800-280-5362
E-Mail: info@graypanthers.org
Web Site: www.graypanthers.org

Gray Panthers is an advocacy and educational organization working for social change by addressing issues such as national health care, jobs, social security, housing, sustainable environment, education, and peace. There are state and local chapters that organize both young and old to work together in addressing Gray Panther issues.

The National Council on Aging
409 3rd Street, S.W., Suite 200
Washington, D.C. 20024
202-479-1200
E-Mail: info@ncoa.org
Web Site: www.ncoa.org

The National Council on Aging (NCOA)—a private, nonprofit organization—serves as a resource for information, training, technical assistance, advocacy, and leadership in all aspects of aging. NCOA seeks to promote the well-being and contributions of older persons and to enhance the field of aging. NCOA believes in the development of innovative methods of meeting the needs of older people.

Older Women's League (OWL)
666 11ᵗʰ Street, N.W., Suite 700
Washington, D.C. 20001
202-783-6686. OWL "PowerLine": 202-783-6689.
Chapter Information: 800-825-3695
OWL is a national organization addressing the special concerns and needs of women as they age. OWL works forcefully to enable its members to achieve economic and social equality for its constituents and to improve the image and status of midlife and older women. OWL holds conferences and programs that provide one-on-one interaction between members and decision-makers in both government and business. The OWL PowerLine gives callers a summary of congressional actions, Supreme Court rulings, government agency reports, and selected press conferences.

This Resource Directory was compiled with assistance from the Administration on Aging's (AoA) web site: (www.aoa.dhhs.gov/aoa/DIR/105.html). Many of the descriptions of the listed organizations were supplied by the AoA staff.

Major Resources on the Web

www.nih.gov
"nih" stands for the "National Institutes of Health", a 75-building "campus" of health institutes, created by Congress over the years, spearheading major research

into the nation's major diseases and health conditions, located in Bethesda, Maryland, near to Washington, DC.

www.cdc.gov
"cdc" stands for the "Centers for Disease Control,"now known as the Centers for Disease Control and Prevention. Located in Atlanta, GA, the CDC is the nation's major medical "detective" on the epidemiology of mysterious outbreaks and the major locus of the nation's health statistics.

www.ncqa.org
This site by the "National Committee for Quality Assurance" offers "reports cards" on health insurers based on zip codes.

www.healthgrades.com
This site (a link from the "National Committee for Quality Assurance" offers "report cards" on hospitals, physicians, nursing homes, home health, hospice and more.

www.merckhomeedition.com
This is an easy guide to otherwise complex diseases. There is a "MediQuiz" testing your knowledge of biology and medical discoveries.

www.americanheart.org
This American Heart Association® site emphasizes warning signs of heart disease and stroke, and invites you to take a quiz on "risk assessment" to see how you fare. Try, also, www.cancer.org (the American Cancer Society) and www.diabetes.org (the American Diabetes Association).

www.mayoclinic.com
This is where you can "talk" to the experts at The Mayo Clinic in Rochester, Minnesota — one of the oldest, most respected clinics combining medical research and clinical practice in the nation. The Mayo web site also provides links to other major medical research organizations and medical centers.

www.medlineplus.gov
This site, a service of the National Library of Medicine and the National Institutes of Health, offers the latest information on prescription medications.

www.nlm.nih.gov
This National Library of Medicine site offers access to over 11 million articles from recognized medical journals in the organization's database.

www.fda.gov
This Food and Drug Administration site is the most current resource on approved drugs for indicated medical uses. It is your guide to the safety and efficacy of drugs, cosmetics and foods.

For Government Benefit Inquiries

www.benefitscheckup.org
Created by the National Council on Aging, this unique web site offers "...a service that identifies federal and state assistance programs for older Americans." Simply log on to the web site and follow the instructions.

The site is completely confidential. You do not have to give your name, address, telephone number or social security number—in fact no information with which you could be identified. The questionnaire, of necessity a bit cumbersome, takes 10-15 minutes to complete. The site then explains what benefits you qualify for and how to apply for them.

APPENDIX D

State and Local Organizations

State and Local Commissions on Aging

Almost every state, and many government agencies, have appointed commissions to advise and advocate on issues relating to aging within the states and areas they represent. At the state level, commissioners are appointed by the governor. At the local level, commissioners are often appointed by locally elected governing bodies.

Aging commissions are formal public bodies, subject to all the laws and regulations that apply to any official board. Their meetings must be announced and open to the public. They can schedule witnesses to appear to give testimony, hold conferences under their auspices to highlight issues of concern, and advocate for changes in laws and for funding of programs affecting the elderly.

Advisory Councils

Under the provisions of the Older Americans Act, every Area Agency on Aging must have an advisory council composed mostly of seniors in the geographic area of the agency. These councils are required to meet regularly and, like the commissions, are bound by the rules of a public body. They set their own agenda, but the local area agency director may ask for advice on matters relating to the agency.

In most states there is an organization at the state level made up of the chairs of the local advisory councils. While these groups can add to the advocacy function of the commissions, they meet mostly to compare notes on the matters that they find in common in their local areas. This means that they often find themselves advising state aging commissions on "bottom-up" issues.

Senior Legislatures

Some states have established their own versions of the original Senior Legislature established in California 20 years ago. Senior legislators (senators and assembly members, mirroring the State Legislature) are elected in each Area Agency on Aging locale. They meet once a year in a weeklong session. Prior to the meeting, legislators submit their ideas for bills to be deliberated and voted on at the session. Committees are appointed to consider and amend the bills and recommend action to the full body.

The recommended bills are voted on in each house and transmitted for consideration by the other house. Bills that are approved by both houses are then given a priority (also by votes). The result is a list of the ten most important issues affecting aging for that year. The list is published and given to the regularly elected members of the legislature and the governor, and members of the Senior Legislature "lobby" for their ten priorities.

State Associations of Area Agencies on Aging

It is almost a given that the directors of the local Area Agencies on Aging form a statewide group, not only to discuss common problems and issues, but also to address matters that concern the state unit on aging, the legislature, and the governor.

In most states, the agency directors are a major influence, for they receive funding from the federal and state governments and are responsible for carrying out aging programs. Agency directors are the managers and coordinators of the programs required by law, and they must contract for those services in strict accord with public laws and regulations—and, of course, be audited to see that their tasks have been done correctly.

Provider Associations

Closely allied with the agency directors are those organizations that provide services under contract. For example, adult day health care programs are provided by nonprofit groups composed of experts in their field. These local providers often have their own statewide associations that, in turn, interact with the directors, the state unit on aging, and the commissions. The providers are free, of course, to advocate for their own agendas, which may not always agree with the others, particularly when it comes to funding.

Advocacy Coalitions

When all these groups combine on any one issue or group of issues, their effectiveness as advocates increases tremendously. Usually, the need felt by all groups has to supercede the need of individual groups. For example, in the budget year 1998-99 in California, there had not been any budget increases in nine years.

Yet the legislature and the governor had just agreed, the year before, to a major reauthorization (and reform) of the Older Californians Act. The commitment to the new Act was political mantra for everyone, so the following year a classic coalition formed, called the Integrated Advocacy Coalition, to advocate for the dollars to at least partially fulfill the promises of the new Act. It worked!

Citizens' Councils

In many states, there are advocacy councils working on behalf of seniors and the elderly. These councils were formed by interest groups to add voice and concern regarding aging-related issues. Many of these groups date back further than government agencies serving the elderly and may, in fact, have "been at the table" when Congressman Claude Pepper was initiating what became the Older Americans Act.

One example is the Congress of California Seniors, which sprung from the traditional labor movement many years ago. Just as organized labor represented the interests of its active members, so also did it advocate for its retirees. To do that the Congress was established, led by retired labor leaders and often funded by the industries in which their members worked. These groups, through meetings and conferences, develop priorities and "lobby" them aggressively. They, too, can form broader coalitions to garner legislative support for common objectives.

BIBLIOGRAPHY

A To Zzzz Guide To Better Sleep, Washington, DC: The Better Sleep Council, c/o Ogilvy Public Relations Worldwide, 1901 L Street, N.W., Washington, DC, 20036 (www.bettersleep.org), 2000.

Anderson, Bob, *Stretching: For Everyday Fitness and for Running, Tennis, Racquetball, Cycling, Swimming, Golf and Other Sports,* Bolinas, CA, Shelter Publications, Inc., 1980.

Barnard, Neal, M.D., *Food for Life,* New York, Harmony Books, 1993.

Beers, Mark H., M.D., and Urice, Stephen K.,Ph.D., J.D. *Aging in Good Health: A Complete, Essential Medical Guide for Older Men and Women and their Families.* New York: Simon & Schuster (Pocket Books), 1995.

Bostwick, David G., and MacLennan, Gregory T., and Thayne R. Larson, *Prostate Cancer: What Every Man–And His Family–Needs To Know.* New York: Villard Press, 1996.

Braddock, Clarence H., III, M.D., M.P.H., and Edwards, Kelly A., M.A., and Hasenberg, Nicole M., M.P.H., and Laidley, Tracy L., M.D., M.P.H., and Levinson, Wendy, M.D., "Informed Decision Making in Outpatient Practice: Time to Get Back to Basics," *Journal of the American Medical Association (JAMA), Vol. 282, No. 24, pp. 2313-2320,* Chicago, The American Medical Association, Dec. 22/29, 1999.

Brooks, David, *Bobos in Paradise: The New Upper Class and How They Got There,* New York: Simon & Schuster, Inc., 2000.

Brown, Janelle, "Shopping On-Line," *Salon Technologies,* Pembroke Pines, FL: Health & Beauty Magazine, 1999.

Burdett, Bob, "What Now?," *New York Times National Report,* New York: The New York Times, 2000.

Campbell, Joseph with Bill Moyers, *The Power of Myth.* New York, Doubleday Publishing/ Random House West, 1988.

Caregiver Pocket Reference, The Prescott, AZ Adult Care Services, Inc., 844 Sunset Avenue, Prescott, AZ 86305, May, 2000.

Davies, Robertson, *Fifth Business,* New York: Viking Penguin Books, Penguin/Putnam, Inc., 1977.

Diabetes Mellites Reference Guide, 6th Edition. Lexington, KY, American Board of Family Practice, 2228 Young Drive, Lexington, KY 40505-4294 (www.abfp.org), 1997.

Diagnostic and Statistical Manual of Mental Disorders (DSM-IV,) 4th Edition, Washington, DC, American Psychiatric Association, 1400 K Street, N.W., Washington, DC 20005 (www.psych.org), 1994.

DoAble Renewable Home, The: Making Your Home Fit Your Needs, Washington, DC, AARP, 601 E Street, N.W., Washington, DC 20049 (www.aarp.org), 2000.

Donnelly, Brian, "A Mature-Market Designer's Path To Becoming A Manufacturer," *Aging Today*. San Francisco: American Society on Aging (ASA), May/June, 2000.

Dorland's Medical Dictionary, Philadelphia: W.B. Saunders Company, 1994.

Dychtwald, Ken, and Flower, Joe, *Age Wave*. Los Angeles: Jeremy P. Tarcher, Inc., 1989.

Eaton, Betty Sue, *Listening to the Garden Grow: Finding Miracles in Daily Life*. Walpole, NH: Stillpoint Publishing, 1996.

Ettinger, Walter H., Jr., M.D., and Mitchell, Brenda S., Ph. D., and Blair, Steven N., PED., *Fitness After 50: It's Never Too Late To Start*, Pasadena, CA, Beverly Cracom Publications, 1996.

Executive Office of the President, The White House, *Patients' Bill of Rights: Executive Memorandum* (signed by former President Bill Clinton on February 20, 1998), Washington, DC, The President's Advisory Commission on Consumer Protection and Quality in the Health Care Industry, 1998.

Executive Office of the President, The White House, The President's Council on Physical Fitness and Sports, *Walking for Exercise and Pleasure* (a pamphlet.) Washington, DC, The President's Council on Physical Fitness and Sports, 1996.

Fact Sheet: "Grandparents as Parents," Washington, DC: Generations United, 122 C Street, N.W., Suite #820, Washington, DC 20001 (www.gu.org), 2001.

Fact Sheet: "Heart & Stroke Statistical Update," Dallas, TX: American Heart Association, 7272 Greenville Avenue, Dallas, TX 75231 (www.americanheart.org), 1999.

Fact Sheet: "New Facts About... Falls And Mobility Disorders in Older Adults," Santa Monica, CA, RAND/Pfizer U.S. Pharmaceuticals, The RAND Corporation, 1700 Main Street, P.O. Box 2138, Santa Monica, CA 90407-2138 (www.rand.org), February, 2000.

Fact Sheet: "New Facts About...Pressure Ulcers in Older Adults," Santa Monica, CA: RAND/Pfizer U.S. Pharmaceuticals, The RAND Corporation, 1700 Main Street, P.O. Box 2138, Santa Monica, CA 90407-2138 (www.rand.org), February, 1999.

Fisher, Stephen, *Colon Cancer and the Polyps Connection.* Tucson, AZ: Fisher Books, 1995.

Flu (a booklet), Bethesda, MD, The National Institute of Allergy and Infectious Diseases, NIAID Office of Communications and Public Liaison, Building 31, Room 7A-50, 31 Center Drive MSC 2520, Bethesda, MD 20892-2520 (www.niaid.gov), 2000.

Foos-Graber, Anna, *Deathing,* York Beach, ME, Nicholas-Hays, Inc., 1989.

Framingham Osteoarthritis Study, The. Santa Monica, CA, RAND and Pfizer U.S. Pharmaceuticals, The RAND Corporation, 1700 Main Street, P.O. Box 2138, Santa Monica, CA 90407-2138 (www.rand.org), 2000.

Getting Fit Your Way: A Self-Paced Fitness Guide. Baltimore: Maryland Department of Health and Mental Hygiene (and the Maryland Army National Guard), Office of Public Affairs, 201 West Preston Street, Baltimore, MD 21201 (www.dhmh.state.md.us), 1983.

Glasser, William M.D., *Choice Theory: A New Psychology of Personal Freedom,* New York: HarperCollins Publishers, 1998.

Goals of Treatment: In Therapy for Diabetes Millitus and Related Disorders, 3rd Edition, Alexandria, VA, American Diabetes Association, 1701 North Beauregard Street, Alexandria, VA 22311 (www.diabetes.org), 1997.

Goldman, Connie, *Tending The Earth, Mending The Spirit: The Healing Gifts of Gardening,* Center City, MN: Hazelden Foundation, 2000.

Gregg, Judd, and Breaux,John, and Kolbe, Jim and Stenholm, Charles W.,"A Look at The Future of Social Security: Building A New Engine For The Old Model," *Outlook Section, 6/7/98.* Washington, DC: The Washington Post, 1998.

Hillman, James, *The Soul's Code: In Search of Character and Calling,* New York: Doubleday Publishing/Random House West, 1996.

Hormone Replacement Therapy: Facts To Help You Decide, Washington, DC, AARP Women's Initiative, 601 E Street, N.W., Washington, DC 20049 (www.aarp.org), 2000.

Hormone Replacement Therapy, Preventing Osteoporosis and The Menopause Years, Washington, DC: The American College of Obstetricians and Gynocologists, 409–12th Street, S.W., P.O. Box 96920, Washington, DC 20090-6920 (www.acog.org), 2000.

"Mini-Mental State: A Practical Method for Grading the Cognitive State of Patients for the Clinician," *Journal of Psychiatric Research, 12(3): 189-198.* Boston: Mini-Mental LLC, 1975.

Jung, Carl with Aneila Jaffe, *Memories, Dreams, Reflections* (revised biography), New York, Pantheon Books, 1973.

Kinship Care Resource Book, The. San Jose, CA, Grandparent Caregiver Resource Center, Catholic Charities of Santa Clara County, 2625 Zanker Road, San Jose, CA 95134, 2000.

Kubler-Ross, Elisabeth, *Death: The Final Stage of Growth.* Englewood Cliffs, NJ, Prentice-Hall, 1975.

Lyder, C., "The Pressure Ulcer Challenge: Balancing Cost and Quality," Washington, DC: The National Pressure Ulcer Advisory Panel, 1998.

"Making Sense of Social Security" (folder), *Americans Discuss Social Security,* Philadelphia, The Pew Charitable Trusts, 1 Commerce Square, 2005 Market Street, Suite #1700, Philadelphia, PA 19103, 1998.

Nash, J. Madeline, "The Estrogen Dilemma," Vol. 155, No. 5, 2/7/00. New York: *Time* Magazine, 2000.

Northrup, Christiane, M.D., *Women's Bodies, Women's Wisdom.* New York: Bantam/Dell Publishing Group, 1998.

Older Americans and Cardiovascular Diseases: Biostatistical Fact Sheets. Dallas, TX: American Heart Association, 7272 Greenville Avenue, Dallas, TX 75231 (www.americanheart.org), 1999.

Ornish, Dean, M.D., *Dr. Dean Ornish's Program For Reversing Heart Disease.* New York: Ballentine Books, 1991.

Ovarian Cancer Special Supplement. New York: Harper's Bazaar, 1999

"Payroll Taxes," Cover Story, 9/24/99. *USA Today.* Arlington, VA, Gannett Publishing Co., 1999.

Pearson, Carol S. Ph.D., *The Hero Within: Six Archetypes We Live By*, Third Edition. San Francisco: HarperSanFrancisco/HarperCollins Publishers, 1998.

Perls, Thomas T., M.D., *Living To 100 Life Expectancy Calculator* (www.livingto100.com) or (www.beeson.org and click on "What is Your Life Expectancy"), The New England Centenarian Study. Boston: The Beeson Organization, 1999.

Peterson, Peter G. *Will America Grow Up Before It Grows Old: How The Coming Social Security Crisis Threatens You, Your Family and Your Country,* New York: Random House, 1996.

Porter, Eleanor, "Share Your Life Story, Baby," *New York Times National Report,* New York: The New York Times, 2000.

Prevention Monograph (pressure ulcers), Washington, DC, The National Pressure Ulcer Advisory Panel (NPUAP), c/o SUNY at Buffalo, Beck Hall, 3435 Main Street, Buffalo, NY 14214 (advisory to the Agency for Healthcare Research and Quality (AHRQ), 2101 East Jefferson Street, Rockville, MD 20852 (www.ahrq.gov), 2000.

Pynoos, Jon and Cohen, Evelyn, *Home Safety Guide for Older People: Check It Out/Fix It Up,* Washington, DC: Serif Press, Inc., 2000.

Regnier, Prof. Victor A., FAIA, *Assisted Living Housing For The Elderly: Design Innovations from the United States and Europe,* New York: John A. Wiley & Sons, Inc., 1994.

Rottenberg, Dan, *The Inheritor's Handbook: A Definitive Guide for Beneficiaries.* New York: Bloomberg Press, 1998.

Rubenstein, L.Z,. and Josephson, K.R., and Robbins, A.S., *Falls in the Nursing Home,* New York: Springer Publishing Co., Inc., 1998.

Schechter-Shalomi, Zalman, Rabbi, with Miller, Ronald S., *From Ageing To Sage-ing.* New York, Warner Books, Inc., 1995.

Silverstone, Barbara and Hyman, Helen Kandel, "Facing Up To Feelings," *You and Your Aging Parents, A Guide To Understanding Emotional, Physical and Financial Needs.* Mount Vernon, NY, Consumers' Union Edition (by permission of Pantheon Books,) 1978, 1982.

Sleep Book, The, Washington, DC, AARP, 601 E Street, N.W., Washington, DC 20049 (www.aarp.org), 2000.

Spoelhof, G.D., and Ide, K., "Pressure Ulcers in Nursing Home Patients," Chicago, *American Family Physician*, 1993.

State of California, Department of Consumer Affairs, Medical Board of California, "Guidelines on Prescribing," *Action Report* (newsletter.) Sacramento, CA, Medical Board of California, 1426 Howe Avenue, Sacramento, CA 95825 (www.medbd.ca.gov), 1994,

State of Oklahoma, Department of Human Services, The Aging Services Division and The Division of Children and Family Services, *Starting Points for Grandparents Raising Grandchildren,* Oklahoma City, OK, Department of Human Services, 2400 North Lincoln Boulevard, P.O. Box 25352, Oklahoma City, OK 73125 (www.okdhs.org), 1999.

Thomas, William H., M.D., *Life Worth Living: How Someone You Love Can Still Enjoy Life in a Nursing Home,* Acton, MA: Wanderwyk & Burnham, 1997.

Tilberis, Liz, *No Time To Die,* Boston, Little, Brown, Inc., 1998.

Tindell, Reverand Charles, *Seeing Beyond The Wrinkles: Stories of Ageless Courage, Humor and Faith.* Northridge, CA: Studio 4 Productions, 1998.

U.S. Consumer Product Safety Commission, *Safety for Older Consumers,* Washington, DC: U.S. Consumer Product Safety Commission, 2000.

U.S. Department of Agriculture, Human Nutrition Information Service, *Dietary Guidelines for Americans,* Washington, DC: U.S. Dept. of Agriculture, 1995.

U.S. Department of Agriculture, Human Nutrition Information Service, *Food Guide Pyramid: A Guide to Daily Food Choices.* Washington, DC, U.S. Department of Agriculture, 1992.

U.S. Department of Agriculture, Human Nutrition Information Service, *Good Source of Nutrients.* Washington, DC, Home and Garden Bulletin No. 252, U.S. Department of Agriculture, 1992.

U.S. Department of Health and Human Services, Administration on Aging, (www.aoa.dhhs.gov, scroll down, click on "AoA Fact Sheets").

U.S. Department of Health and Human Services, Administration on Aging, National Institute on Aging and the National Aeronautics and Space Administration, *Exercise: A Guide from The National Institute on Aging and the National Aeronautics and Space Administration,* Washington, DC: Information Center, National Institute on Aging, 2000.

U.S. Department of Health and Human Services, Administration on Aging, National Institute on Aging, *Shots for Safety* (a bulletin), Washington, DC: The National Institute on Aging, 2000.

U.S. Department of Health and Human Services, Centers for Disease Control and Prevention, *Immunization of Adults: A Call To Action.* Atlanta, GA, The Centers for Disease Control and Prevention, 2000.

U.S. Dept. of Health and Human Services, Centers for Disease Control and Prevention, *National Nursing Home Survey.* Atlanta, GA, National Center for Health Statistics, Centers for Disease Control and Prevention, U.S. Government Printing Office, S/N 017-022-01481-5, 1995.

U.S. Dept. of Health and Human Services, Centers for Disease Control and Prevention, National Center for Chronic Disease Prevention and Health Promotion, *Physical Activity and Health: A Report of the Surgeon General,* Atlanta, GA, Centers for Disease Control and Prevention, 1996.

U.S. Department of Health and Human Services, Centers for Disease Control and Prevention, National Center for Health Statistics, *Deaths: Final Data for 1997, National Vital Statistics Reports, Vol. 47, No. 19.* Atlanta, GA, Centers for Disease Control and Prevention, 1999.

U.S. Dept. of Health, Education and Welfare, Public Health Service, Office of the Assistant Secretary for Health and Surgeon General, *Healthy People: The Surgeon General's Report on Health Promotion and Disease Prevention,* Washington, DC: U.S. Government Printing Office, DHEW Publication No. (PHS) 79-55071, 1979. (Part of the *Healthy People* series.)

U.S. Dept. of Health and Human Services, Public Health Service, Office of the Assistant Secretary for Health, *Healthy People 2000, National Health Promotion and Disease Prevention Objectives,* Washington, DC, U.S. Government Printing Office, DHHS Publication No. (PHS) 91-50213, 1991. (Part of the *Healthy People* series.)

U.S. Dept. of Health and Human Services, Public Health Service, Office of the Assistant Secretary for Health, *Healthy People 2010: Understanding and Improving Health,* Washington, DC, U.S. Government Printing Office, DHHS Publication No. (PHS) 98-1256, 2000. (Part of the *Healthy People* series.)

U.S. Department of Health and Human Services, National Institute of Mental Health, *Depression in Primary Care... Clinical Practice Guideline* (a study), Washington, DC, National Institute of Mental Health, 1993.

U.S. Dept. of Health and Human Services, Public Health Service, Office of the Assistant Secretary for Health, *Promoting Health/Preventing Disease: Objectives for the Nation.* Washington, DC, U.S. Government Printing Office, (published in November, 1980, but not available in print); available in major libraries; part of the *Healthy People* series.)

U.S. Social Security Administration (Office of Public Inquiries, 6401 Security Boulevard, Room 4-C-5 Annex, Baltimore, MD 21235-6401 [www.ssa.gov]).

Social Security Retirement Benefits (#05-10035.) Washington, DC, Social Security Administration, 2000.

Social Security–Understanding The Benefits (#05-10024.) Washington, DC, Social Security Administration, 2000.

"Volunteer Participation in California, A Report on," *Aging Network News.* Sacramento, CA, California Department of Aging, 1600 K Street, Sacramento, CA 95814 (www.aging.state.ca.us), 1998.

Waggoner, Glen, "Getting Tough With Telemarketers," *Modern Maturity*, July-August, 1999. Washington, DC, AARP, 1999.

Waid, Mary Onnis, *Brief Summaries of Medicare and Medicaid, Title XVIII and Title XIX of the Social Security Act (July 31, 1998),* Washington, DC, Office of the Actuary, Health Care Financing Administration, U.S. Department of Health and Human Services, 1998.

"Watching for Warning Signs" (Alzheimer's Disease), January 31, 2000, New York: *Newsweek* Magazine, 2000.

Webster's New World Dictionary and Thesaurus, New York, MacMillan/Simon & Schuster, Inc., 1996.

Welwood, John, *Toward A Psychology of Awakening.* Boston: Shambhala Publications, 2000.

Weston, Liz Pulliam, "Most Households Not Saving Enough for Retirement, Analysis Shows," *Business Section, 4/27/00.* Los Angeles: The Los Angeles Times, 2000.

White, John, *A Practical Guide To Death and Dying.* Wheaton, IL: Theosophical Publishing House, 1980.

Zweig, Connie, Ph.D., and Wolf, Steve, Ph.D., *Romancing The Shadow: Illuminating The Dark Side of the Soul.* New York: Ballantine Books, 1997.

INDEX